CARING FOR THE DYING PATIENT AND THE FAMILY

Edited by Joy Robbins, BA, SRN, SCM, RNT
Senior Tutor, St Joseph's Hospice, London

Harper & Row, Publishers
London

Cambridge
Mexico City
New York
Philadelphia

San Francisco
São Paulo
Singapore
Sydney

First published 1983
Reprinted 1987

Harper & Row Ltd
28 Tavistock Street
London WC2E 7PN

British Library Cataloguing in Publication Data
Care of the dying patient and the family.
1. Terminal care 2. Death
I. Robbins, Joy
362.1   R762.8
ISBN 0-06-318249-1

Typeset by Bookens, Saffron Walden, Essex
Printed by Butler and Tanner, Frome, Somerset

CARING FOR THE DYING PATIENT
AND THE FAMILY

CONTENTS

PREFACE

When this book was first suggested very little had been produced for British nurses which encompassed practical as well as philosophical aspects of care for dying people and their families. Several publications of this nature have now appeared, and we are pleased to offer another, similar in aims but different in format. Most of the contributors are either working at St Joseph's Hospice or have done so in the past. All, however, write from an experience of many different health care settings as well.

This multiprofessional approach strengthened the main aim of the book, namely, to further the understanding of nurses regarding the needs of human beings at the end of life, whether the nurse is working in a hospital, hospice or other institution, or in a patient's home. It is hoped that the student nurse will find the book useful as a comprehensive text throughout her training. We have also the trained nurse in mind who could use the book as a basis for further study, particularly as a post-basic student in one of the clinical courses approved by the National Boards. The references provided at the end of each chapter indicate an awareness that no one book of this size can give equal emphasis to all aspects of care, or do perfect justice to any. The book should also be of interest to all those in other professions who are closely involved with nurses in the caring team.

ACKNOWLEDGEMENTS

My task as editor would have been impossible without the help and guidance of many people. My sincere thanks are due to the contributors who wrote the book with me, willingly co-operating and spending a considerable amount of time outside their working day. Cathy Peck, Senior Editor of Harper and Row Publishers, was a constant source of encouragement and advice, especially in times of frustration, and I am greatly indebted to her.

I am grateful to Dr J Hanratty for his encouragement and advice.

The initial acceptance of the challenge to produce the book is due to Sister Paula (then Matron of St Joseph's Hospice) and I am honoured that she entrusted me with the editorship. Finally, I am mindful of uncounted numbers of dying patients and their families in whom those who wrote this book found their inspiration.

Joy Robbins

NOTE: All royalties from sales of this book will go to St Joseph's Hospice.

LIST OF CONTRIBUTORS

Sister Marcella Cassells, SRN
Ward Sister, St Joseph's Hospice, London

Peggy Collinge, SRN, RSCN, SCM, RCNT, DipN (Lond)
Clinical Teacher, Queen Elizabeth Hospital for Sick Children, London

John Collins, MB, ChB, DRCOG
GP trainee (formerly Macmillan Service, St Joseph's Hospice, London)

Harriet Copperman, SRN, SCM, NDN Cert
Sister, Support/Symptom Control Team, Royal Free Hospital, London
(formerly Macmillan Service, St Jospeh's Hospice, London)

Sister Catherine Egan, SRN
Ward Sister, St Joseph's Hospice, London

Sister Paula Gleeson
Formerly Matron, St Joseph's Hospice, London

James P Hanratty, MB, ChB, MRCGP
Medical Director, St Joseph's Hospice, London

Marion Judd, MNZSP, SPR
Physiotherapist, Macmillan Service, St Joseph's Hospice, London

Margaret Linton, SRN, SCM
Midwifery Sister, City & Hackney Health District, London

Sister Finbarr Malone, SRN
Deputy Matron, St Joseph's Hospice, London

Sister Helena Marie McGilly, SRN, SCM, DN Cert
Director of Nursing, Macmillan Service, St Joseph's Hospice, London

Paul McGinn
Priest in Charge, Church of St John the Baptist, Hackney, London
(Formerly Chaplain, St Joseph's Hospice, London)

Beryl Munns, MSc, BA, SRN, SCM, QN, HV Cert
Nursing Officer (Teaching/Research), St Joseph's Hospice, London

Sister Antonia O'Connor, SRN
Ward Sister (formerly Macmillan Service), St Joseph's Hospice, London

Sister Micheline O'Donnell
Ward Sister, St Margaret's Hospice, Glasgow

Jenny Pardoe, MA, CQSW
Director of Social Work, Macmillan Service, St Joseph's Hospice, London

Katie M Pfister, SRN, SCM, RNT
Nurse Tutor, St Joseph's Hospice, London

Joy Robbins, BA, SRN, SCM, RNT
Senior Tutor, St Joseph's Hospice, London

Elizabeth D Stewart, SRN, RSCN, SCM, RCNT
Nursing Officer, Queen Elizabeth Hospital for Sick Children, London

Barbara Saunders, SRN, RCNT
Clinical Nurse Adviser, Terminal Care Support Team, St Thomas's Hospital, London

Sister Mary Wynne
Sister in Charge, Recreational Therapy Department, St Joseph's Hospice, London

NOTE: The title Sister denotes members of the Congregation of the Irish Sisters of Charity

CHAPTER 1

ATTITUDES TO DEATH AND DYING
JOY ROBBINS

Some common attitudes to death

Thoughts about death arouse many emotions, especially that of fear, when there is a personal connotation. We can speak impartially about the subject unless it is about our own death or that of a close relative or friend. From the earliest times man has found a fascination, mixed with awe, at the mystery of death. We find it difficult to accept that our lives and very personalities will one day come to a halt. The physical fact of a lifeless body can be seen – but where is the person? Attitudes are influenced by cultural traditions and the possession of a religious faith with a promise of life after death and continuation of a personal life in some form. In modern society many people profess to discount any such belief, or to be uncertain of its validity. This will have a bearing on the attitudes of the dying person and of those close to him*; it will also be a factor to be kept in mind by the caring team. Age plays a part in determining attitudes; it is natural that thoughts of personal death will present more often to elderly people than to young healthy adults.

During the latter half of this century, there has been increasing aware-ness that much unnecessary suffering both physical and psychological has been caused to many dying people and their families because of in-

---

*For the sake of conciseness, the patient is generally referred to as 'he' and the nurse as 'she'.

adequate help by professional carers, and the artificial barriers erected by contemporary society to hide the facts of death and dying.

The historical perspective

Since knowledge and perception affect attitudes, it is instructive to compare the life span of human beings in this and other Western countries before and after the Industrial Revolution. Although there is no systematic data available, it is known that about 200 years ago most people died at what would now be regarded as the 'prime of life', or in infancy when death rates were particularly high.

By 1840, the population in most European countries had a life expectancy of 40+ years; by 1930 this was 60+ years, and by 1950 had risen to over 70 years. This dramatic change (the infant mortality rate fell remarkably) arose mainly because of over-all improvement in living standards – better housing, sanitation and agricultural methods resulting in more food being available. The rapid advances in twentieth-century medicine further reduced the mortality rate. Thus an environment of 'controlled mortality' now prevails, and this has produced a very different life style from that in previous centuries. Family size is smaller, by choice, and great emotional and financial resources are invested in the children because they, like their parents, are expected to have a long life. More time is devoted to formal education and much energy and money is devoted to research and therapy aimed at curing disease and further extending life. The remoteness of death diminishes the orientation towards religious explanations of the ultimate end.

Causes and location of death

In Western society the main causes of death are degenerative diseases, particularly of the cardiovascular system, malignant diseases and accidents. This last category leads to the fact that in our present century, unnatural forms of death have increased dramatically, including homicide, self-destruction and road traffic accidents.

Regrettably, human beings have always killed each other, but it is the sheer size of the phenomenon that is startling. Apart from the two world wars, the Nazi gas chambers (killing 6 million Jews and other 'undesirables'), the explosion of the atom bombs at Hiroshima, and international terrorism are global reminders of the contemporary face of death. The tensions of modern life have contributed to the marked rise in suicides in developed countries. Yet Western society now finds public execution revolting and indeed in the main has rejected imposition of the death penalty for serious crime. Such are the complex issues which are present in the development of cultural attitudes.

Whereas in the past most people died at home, a shift has occurred in this century, removing death from the home into an institution. About 60% of deaths in this country occur in general hospitals. This tends to isolate further the dying person from the rest of society, and the fact of death as a natural part of everyday life. More people grow up from childhood to maturity without witnessing the natural death of a close relative, although paradoxically much entertainment for adults and children concerns killings. Bereavement may be harder to bear because many of the former rituals of mourning, such as a church funeral, wearing black and visits to the home of the bereaved by friends and neighbours, are less common, and manifestations of grief are less open and acceptable.

Attitudes of dying people

When a person is actually dying many thoughts and emotions may occupy the mind. The nature of those is well recognized and documented; it should be realized that every human being will react differently and emotions will often be mingled and change from one extreme to the other quite frequently if dying is gradual. Elizabeth Kubler-Ross (1970 and 1982) has by her research provided a major contribution in this field.

The following emotions will be witnessed in dying patients but not necessarily in any particular order or all in one person.

Anxiety and fear

The instinctive fear of approaching dissolution may be observed if the patient suspects that his illness is a fatal one, and has not been able to come to terms with it. The facial expression will be anxious and restlessness and tension apparent. On the other hand, patients may conceal their fears, perhaps because they cannot face them, or because they find that no opportunity is given to discuss them with a sympathetic listener. Some of the sources of the fears may be tangible, such as possible effects of their disease. For instance, a patient with malignant growth in the thorax may fear that he will suffocate. The patient who is aware of increasing girth and discomfort from an abdominal mass may have a vivid picture of bursting open. A husband or wife may be very anxious about the welfare – financial and otherwise – of the spouse and any children who will be left alone after the death. Patients may be frightened of being left alone, or of dying alone whilst asleep.

Depression and sadness

These are very understandable reactions in a patient who has had a long illness with possible painful and protracted treatment, particularly for cancer. In the terminal stage of his illness, and with increasing sensations of weakness he may feel that all the endurance of such treatment was futile. Anger and resentment – 'Why me?' – may merge with depression, and if a sense of withdrawal by relatives and staff unable to cope with their own painful emotion is added, the patient may well find the situation intolerable. Inadequate relief of symptoms is itself an important cause of misery and depression. These facts should lead nurses and doctors to reflect seriously on their responsibilities and practice in the care of dying patients.

Denial and acceptance

Considerable research has taken place into the insight of dying patients about their true condition and prognosis, and those with experience will testify how difficult it is in many cases to be sure of what the patient understands and believes. It is generally accepted among those working closely with dying patients that the patient's right to indicate whether he wishes to discuss his illness in depth or not must be respected. A number of research projects, such as those undertaken by Elizabeth Kubler-Ross (1970 and 1982), show that many patients do realize that they are dying, through their own intuition. Sometimes a patient may have requested a frank discussion and have apparently understood that his life span is expected to be a short one. Other emotions may then intervene, such as hope that the doctor may be mistaken – the patient practising a denial of the information given, as a defence mechanism. Younger patients may go through a distressing phase of struggling against the inevitable outcome, with bitterness and resentment.

Fortunately most dying patients become peaceful and calm during their last hours, many during the final weeks, providing that sufficient help has been given in total care, that is: physical, mental, social and spiritual.

The patient and the family

While there is still some uncertainty whether a person's illness, although grave, is a mortal one, the patient or more likely the family may search frantically for a cure, seeking further opinions from more than one doctor or trying unorthodox forms of healing. Those with a religious faith will pray earnestly for a cure, and may take the patient to a shrine such as Lourdes. The professional team should respect these actions, and when there is final realization and acceptance of approaching death, the family is often comforted by the thought that they have done all they could for their loved one in an effort to preserve his life.

Some people may struggle against their inevitable progress towards death until the very end, and it will be distressing for those caring for such patients to witness their fear and lack of peace. John Hinton in his book *Dying* (1972) suggests that the person in this condition may need the hope and refusal to surrender, rather than the desolation of no hope at all.

In contrast, a peaceful acceptance of death is common among the elderly, who may find particular comfort in the continuity of their family life in their children and grandchildren. For those who have made careful preparation for death in the matter of their personal affairs, this in itself can give an emotional satisfaction and relaxation.

The relevance of religious belief to dying people is, of course, important. A research study into a group of dying patients (Hinton 1972) revealed that those who had a firm religious faith were the most free from anxiety. Those who maintained that they had no religious beliefs also appeared calm during their last illness. The group who showed most anxiety were those who were uncertain and wavering in their belief in and practice of a religious faith.

One attitude of close relatives which, though understandable, will cause sadness to the dying person is an emotional withdrawal at the very time when he most needs companionship and understanding from those he loves. This situation may be due to embarrassment as to how to behave or what to say, or to an increasing sense of grief at the impending separation, which the relative feels unable to share with the dying person.

Close relatives often exhibit some or all of the emotional stages through which the dying person is passing. The sense of loss begins before the actual death and anticipatory grief will be experienced as part of the bereavement process. Such specialists as Doctor Colin Murray-Parkes (1972: introduction and chap. 1) have by their research contributed to a better understanding of bereavement and how families can be helped.

This topic is dealt with in some detail in Chapter 13.

Attitudes of the nurse

Since attitudes are related to behaviour, it is important that the nurse who will care for dying patients and their families recognizes the effect of her personal thoughts and feelings about death – her own and other people's. Nurses, like doctors, are sometimes placed on a pedestal and expected to show supernatural qualities of strength and equability in any situation. They may themselves suppress their own fears and anxieties by erecting barriers in their professional work, allowing only a superficial interaction with their patients – a 'them' and 'us' relationship. Acknowledging a common humanity which includes at times feelings of inadequacy and anxiety, and talking over problems with colleagues, is a sign of growth, not weakness.

The student nurse is usually young and, like her contemporaries, has quite probably never met death and dying at first hand before. Unlike her friends entering other professional trainings or various forms of employment, she must face the sure prospect of intimate contact with dying people, of witnessing the anguish of families facing the loss of a loved one, and of providing the final physical care to the dead body before this is relinquished to the funeral director. It is understandable if the anticipation of these responsibilities may cause some apprehension. Most nurses remember clearly when they first looked upon the face of a dead person and found with relief that the sight was peaceful and not frightening.

Attitudes of respect in handling the body and carrying out Last Offices are well-established at an early stage of training and passed on to junior colleagues by precept and example. Few nurses appear to have lasting difficulties in this sphere, although this refers to death from natural causes, at home or in hospital. The sight and handling of mutilated bodies in war or from major accidents will inevitably be unpleasant and emotionally difficult to manage.

It is in the area of communication with dying patients and grieving relatives that difficulties often occur for the nurse in trying to acquire attitudes that will be of maximum help. It is encouraging to remember that actions speak louder than words, and the nurse who demonstrates gentle, effective physical care for the patient, given in an unhurried manner, or simple courtesy and concern for a tired and anxious relative is communicating a positive and caring attitude. To be prepared to listen with whole-hearted attention and to respond to the best of one's ability, offering to bring a more experienced colleague to continue the dialogue if appropriate, is to give a valuable service.

Because of her unique type of involvement with dying patients, the nurse needs to have a sensible attitude towards her own health, both for self-interest and in order to give of her best to those in her care. This is particularly so where she works exclusively in the field of terminal care. She should have plenty of interests and recreation with friends away from the working environment, as well as family contacts, so that she returns to work refreshed and happy. The ability to convey a warm, positive attitude is an important attribute and helps to surround the patient with a natural, pleasant atmosphere without false brightness and over-optimism.

Possession of a religious faith, or a stable philosophy about the fundamental issues of life and death, helps to provide an inner strength for the nurse which in turn aids her in caring for patients and families in distress.

The nurse may herself have suffered a bereavement and thus have insight into the feelings of a grieving family. Even if she has never lost a close member of her own family, many forms of loss, e.g. loss of self-esteem or a valued possession, or a broken engagement, mirror in some degree the pain of actual bereavement. Reflecting on such experiences can assist in developing helpful attitudes to bereaved relatives, when shared with experienced colleagues.

Death itself is a mystery and one has no personal point of reference, i.e. personal experience. Unfortunately, lack of understanding and avoidance of facing the problem has meant that for many years the fears and loneliness associated with dying have not been openly considered and helped sufficiently by those professional groups, including nurses, who are in the best position to do so. This situation is gradually changing for the better, and continuing education in these matters for all concerned is spreading. By learning from observing more experienced colleagues, by reading from the considerable literature now available, and by overcoming any tendency to avoid dying patients because of painful and inadequate feelings in ourselves, we can demonstrate a more confident attitude to the dying patient in our efforts to make his dying comfortable in body, mind and spirit.

References

Carr, C A (1979) The problem: denial and ambivalence toward death, in H Wass (Editor) Dying – Facing the facts, McGraw-Hill

Hinton, J (1972) Dying, Pelican Books

Kubler-Ross, E (1970) On Death and Dying, Tavistock

Kubler-Ross, E (1982) Living with Death and Dying, Macmillan

Parkes, C Murray (1972) Studies of Grief in Adult Life (introduction and chap. 1), Pelican Books

CHAPTER 2

NURSING ASSESSMENT
JOY ROBBINS

Introduction

It is increasingly accepted by nurses that, in order to provide a high quality of care for a patient, it is valuable to spend time in forming a comprehensive picture of the individual's physical and mental state, to identify potential nursing problems and to plan the care needed on this basis. Obviously, these activities will be sterile unless followed by the actual provision of care and modification of the original plans as appears necessary in order to meet the desired goals as effectively as possible.

These four stages of the nursing process:

assessment of the patient's condition and needs
planning of care
implementation of the plan
evaluation of the effectiveness of the care given

can be applied with considerable benefit to the nursing care of the dying patient and the family

Assessment of the dying patient

It is important to remember that the patient may have one or more problems not directly related to the main diagnosis and causing considerable discomfort and worry. For instance, the patient with advanced breast cancer may also have such problems as toothache, painful corns or joint pains due to arthritis. Just as the doctor should carry out a thorough physical examination and take a careful medical history, so must the nurse make a complete assessment of the patient in order to ascertain the nursing needs.

First meeting with the patient

It is a truism that first impressions are crucial in any situation where two people are hoping to build up a relationship. Unless the dying patient is deeply unconscious, he is also making observations about the nurse at their first meeting. Thus the assessment stage is mutual, although of course from different standpoints.

The nurse's aim is to gather essential information by observation, examination and discussion with the patient in order to plan the best possible nursing. The dying patient's aim, whether formulated or not, is to judge from observing the nurse whether she is interested in him, compassionate, and whether she inspires confidence in her ability to relieve distressing symptoms, which may include fear and loneliness with a longing to find a sympathetic listener.

To gain the patient's co-operation in her assessment of his state, the nurse needs to be aware of these thoughts which may be present in the patient's mind, and to respond in the appropriate way.

The nurse's manner of approach

A recent research study (Ashworth 1980: p. 17) refers to the positive effect on human interaction of physical proximity, eye contact, a friendly tone of voice and conversation about personal topics. The nurse establishing contact with the dying patient can make use of these findings as follows:

1   By sitting close to the patient, by his bed or chair where it is easy to talk face to face. A smile and friendly greeting should be immediate.

2   By attention to the tone of voice and articulation. The patient may not be able to hear well whether through age or weakness, so that a clear, measured mode of speech helps. Courtesy, shown by addressing the patient by his correct title, and warmth of tone imply concern and interest.

3   Touch is a powerful source of social bonding and the nurse should take the patient's hand in the initial greeting. Where it seems helpful, as with a patient who is obviously distressed and anxious, the nurse should not hesitate to hold the patient's hand gently for a time.

These initial steps to establish contact are very important to the dying patient in showing that care will include the unhurried offering of time by his professional carers, especially in being prepared to listen.

Obtaining information

Having established contact, and expended effort in gaining the patient's confidence, the nurse should have a clear idea of the sort of information she needs in order to identify problems and plan the appropriate nursing care. This will be done by asking the patient questions, by observation and examination.

Much has been written in recent years about obtaining a nursing history, and the various ways to do this. Flexibility seems to be the consensus of opinion, and that information by verbal questioning must be obtained gradually over a period of time.

The dying patient may be quite unable to answer any but the minimum of necessary questions, due to weakness, pain, confusion or other distressing symptoms, and the nurse may have to rely on the relatives to supply the necessary information.

Proper recording and reporting of information is as important for the care of this patient as for any other. Whatever the type of nursing history sheet used, it must be a helpful, practical basis for planning the total care of the patient – physical, psychological, social and spiritual. Simplicity is the keynote; an elaborate and time-consuming procedure is not appropriate, particularly as the patient may have a very limited time to live, perhaps only hours.

One factor that is of particular importance for all those caring for the dying patient is the extent of insight that he appears to have into the nature and prognosis of his illness. Today, many patients are well informed as to their diagnosis, and will volunteer this information readily. Indeed, the patient in the terminal stage of congestive heart failure or chronic bronchitis is only too well aware of years of ill health and many forms of treatment. The patient with a malignant disease is also not unlikely to refer to a growth or tumour, or actually to use the word cancer to describe his condition. Assessing whether the patient understands that he is dying is often difficult and needs time for relationships to be established between the patient and his carers. On the other hand, some patients will make their thoughts clear at the outset, in direct statements about their approaching demise, or in a firm optimism about an eventual cure. This information should be recorded in the nursing history sheet whether it has been obtained by the nurse or another colleague, so that all the caring team are aware of the extent of the patient's insight into his condition.

Personal lifestyle   The nurse will need to find out a number of practical details in order to provide the maximum comfort for the patient. These will include sleeping habits, special likes or dislikes in food and drink, recreational interests and any prosthesis worn, such as hearing aid, dentures or spectacles. In enquiring about the patient's religious beliefs, it should be ascertained if he has any special wishes in this respect. Worries may be expressed regarding finance or family welfare, and these should be noted for the attention of the social worker, after assuring the patient that help will be forthcoming.

The help of an interpreter may be needed if the patient does not have a good command of English; otherwise increased anxiety will be an additional burden for the patient, and difficult for the nurse.

Observation of the patient

The nurse can learn much by observing the patient during the initial contact, as the following examples will demonstrate.

Facial expression   This may reflect pain, anxiety, apathy, hostility, depression, one of which will give a clue to underlying problems both physical and psychological. On the other hand, the patient may appear serene and smiling. People may mask their feelings so that superficial observation of the face does not reveal the true state of affairs. It is thus helpful to try and see the patient 'off guard' before or after actually meeting him face to face.

Position in bed/chair   Many dying patients prefer to be out of bed for part of the day and even walking about until weakness overwhelms the power of mobility. Posture can again reveal emotional problems such as depression or anxiety, and certainly pain. The patient may be sitting or lying in an unnatural position with contorted limbs. If walking about, the degree of agility can be noted, and the presence of a limp. The depressed patient may be hunched up, with bent head, or hidden under the bed-clothes. Anxiety or confusion is often accompanied by restlessness and twisting of the hands.

Odour   On approaching the patient, the nurse may be aware of an odour which gives a clue to a particular problem even before close proximity. The smell of faeces or urine alerts one to a situation of incontinence or a badly controlled stoma. The patient may not actually be vomiting at the time, but contamination of personal clothing by vomit on a previous occasion may not have been dealt with adequately and leaves a typical lingering odour. The presence of a fungating wound is not uncommon, especially in advanced breast cancer, and will certainly have unpleasant odour which may be apparent even when the wound is not exposed.

Sounds Respiratory symptoms are common in the dying patient so that the nurse may hear the patient coughing, breathing noisily or, if death is near and secretions are filling the trachea which the patient cannot expel, the so-called 'death rattle'. In listening to the patient, the nurse may notice a speech impediment such as slurring, or hoarseness of voice.

Level of consciousness When first meeting a dying patient, a wide range of mental states will be observed. Some patients remain alert and conscious right up to the last moments before death occurs. This can be the case in the terminal stage of a chronic illness as well as in sudden and unexpected death.

In a chronic illness, most patients lapse into coma during the last few hours if not earlier. A semi-conscious state is common during the last 48 hours, especially during the terminal stage of a malignant disease. The nurse may realize that the patient is confused to some degree and unable to give reliable information by word of mouth.

Physical examination of the patient
This should be done gently and unobtrusively, and starts with the first attempt to make the patient comfortable in bed or chair, and more comprehensively when dealing with the patient's clothing, bedding and skin toilet.

Specific observations will include:

Colour, texture and integrity of skin and mucous membranes.
Presence of swellings in any part of the body.
Oedema or muscle wasting.
Abnormal position of limbs.
Unusual movements such as shaking or trembling.
Incontinence of urine or faeces.
Level of consciousness and orientation.

The nurse will, of course, gain further information from the doctor's findings, such as the result of rectal or vaginal examination, abdominal palpation, and the quality of cardiac and respiratory functions. She should also be aware of the signs of impending death as her first contact with the patient may be at a late stage in the terminal illness (see Chapter 8).

Assessment of the family

All those caring for dying patients testify to the need to consider him as part of the family unit when assessing the situation and planning care. In a paper written about inpatient care of patients with advanced malignant disease, Dr T. S. West actually uses the phrase 'admitting the family' (*in* Saunders 1978).

Further chapters in this book will refer frequently to family members and their needs. With regard to initial assessment and planning of care by the nurse, she will need to show the same alertness as with the patient in observing for signs of anxiety, exhaustion and actual ill health in close members of the family. A methodical history should be taken to obtain the fullest information possible, the family's perception of the patient's problems, and the part they have played so far in caring for him.

A sympathetic, warm approach on the nurse's part lays the foundation for continuing co-operation with those relatives who will either visit the patient in hospice or hospital, or continue to care for him at home. It is also important to plan what action is necessary for the support of the family in co-operation with other colleagues, e.g. doctor, social worker, chaplain.

Where the patient has no living relatives, his professional carers must become his 'family' to some extent.

Conclusion

This chapter has set out the first stages of the process of nursing a dying patient and his family, i.e. assessment. A number of subsequent chapters will deal with establishing nursing goals, giving appropriate care and evaluating its effectiveness. Further chapters have been written by professional colleagues who are experts in other aspects of care, such as medicine and social work. There will be some overlap between all the writers, which will serve to re-inforce important points, and also to reflect the fact that, to be successful, care of the dying patient and his family is a team effort which people share for a common goal: namely death in peace, comfort and dignity.

References

Ashworth, P (1980) Care to Communicate (p. 17), Royal College of Nursing

Lamerton, R (1980) Care of the Dying, Pelican Books

Long, R (1981) Systematic Nursing Care, Faber and Faber

Saunders, C M (ed) (1978) The Management of Terminal Disease, Edward Arnold

West, T S (1978) Inpatient management of advanced malignant disease, (p. 143) in C M Saunders (Editor) The Management of Terminal Disease, Edward Arnold

CHAPTER 3

NURSING AIMS AND GIVING CARE I
SISTER HELENA McGILLY and
SISTER CATHERINE EGAN

Following assessment of the patient and family, it should be possible to identify problems, state the nursing goals and describe how care will be given. Many aspects of nursing care of a dying patient are also applicable to the seriously ill person who is not dying. It is the *special* needs, associated with a number of common problems, that will be considered in this chapter and the following one.

The patient with nausea and vomiting

The patient feels ill and weak, often with dizziness, headaches and sweating. Constant retching may become a nightmare and cause tenderness and a sensation of bruising over the sternum. Vomiting causes mental distress, since the patient feels that it is offensive to others, and diminishes his own self-respect and dignity.

Causes of nausea and vomiting in the dying patient may be one or more of the following:

constipation
radiotherapy
uraemia
electrolyte imbalance, e.g. hypercalcaemia
infections, e.g. urinary infection

gastric irritation, e.g. from a tumour
hepatic metastases
intestinal obstruction
vestibular disturbance
coughing
fear and anxiety

Giving nursing care

Aims of care

1   To help in identifying possible causes of the problem by use of observation.
2   To control the symptoms by administering any prescribed anti-emetic drugs.
3   To improve the patient's comfort by hygiene.
4   To raise the patient's morale.

The patient may have had these distressing symptoms for a prolonged period and needs assurance that immediate action will be taken to relieve his misery. Any cause which has been identified and can be removed should be dealt with. In severe constipation the bowel should be cleared by means of an effective enema or manual removal if faeces are impacted. Drugs suspected of causing nausea and vomiting should be withdrawn. If they are essential they should be given in a form to diminish their nauseating propensity, for instance prednisolone given with an enteric coating. Many of the causes of nausea and vomiting in the dying patient cannot be removed, and therefore the treatment is symptomatic.

The use of anti-emetic drugs is invariably prescribed, and the following are ones which the nurse is likely to administer, and whose action and side-effects she should be familiar with, so that she can help the doctor to assess if the drug itself is suitable and the dosage prescribed is appropriate.

Anti-emetic medications

1   *antihistamines*
cyclizine 50 mg three times a day as tablets or by injection.
promethazine 25 mg three times a day – makes patient rather drowsy.
dimenhydrinate 100 mg three times a day – useful for vestibular type of vomiting but makes patient drowsy.

2   *butyrophenones*
droperidol 10 mg three times a day as tablets or by injection – useful for vomiting after chemotherapy.
haloperidol 0.5–1.5 mg three times a day as tablets, capsules, liquid or in ampoules for injection – continued use causes extrapyramidal effects.

3   *phenothiazines*
prochlorperazine 5–10 mg 4-hourly or three times a day as tablets, syrup, suppositories or in ampoules for injection.
promazine 25 mg three times a day as tablets, suspension or in ampoules for injection.
chlorpromazine – anti-emetic dose is between 10 mg and 25 mg four times a day as tablets, syrup, in ampoules for injection, or as 100 mg suppositories.
methotrimeprazine 25 mg as tablets or injection twice a day – has sedative and analgesic effects as well as being an anti-emetic.

Prolonged or large doses of phenothiazines may produce twitching – dyskinesia – which usually ceases on reducing the dose. The patient may appear to be restless or fidgety. Tardive dyskinesia is a more serious toxic effect and takes the form of persistent uncontrollable grimacing. This does not always cease on withdrawing the drug but it only occurs usually in patients who have been taking phenothiazines for many months or years. Dryness of the mouth may also be caused by phenothiazines but is usually dose-related.

4   *metoclopramide* 5–10 mg three times a day as tablets, syrup or in ampoules for injection. This drug has central and peripheral anti-emetic actions. It accelerates gastric peristalsis and as it also increases the tone of the gastro-oesophageal sphincter it augments gastric emptying. Its action on the chemoreceptor trigger zone has a central anti-emetic effect.
domperidone 10 mg as tablets 4-hourly or in ampoules for intra-muscular or intravenous injection – a dopamine antagonist and also affects gastric motility.

5   *anticholinergics*
hyoscine 0.4 mg by injection – an effective anti-emetic but it causes dry mouth, blurring of vision and drowsiness. It is more useful as a means of drying secretions in the final few hours.

There is no point in using different phenothiazines at the same time but resistant cases may benefit from a combination of prochlorperazine (Stemetil), metoclopramide (Maxolon) and cyclizine. A continuous subcutaneous infusion of one or more of these drugs may be given via the Greaseby Syringe Driver (see p. 75).

Treatment in certain situations

Gastric irritation Magnesium trisilicate mixture 10 ml three times a day; Asilone tablets or suspension; Gaviscon tablets to chew or liquid 10 ml twice a day; Pyrogastrone tablets to chew.

Oesophageal reflux: Mucaine suspension 10 ml before meals; cimetidine 200 mg three times a day and 400 mg at night; Ranitidine 150 mg twice a day.

Hypercalcaemia Occurs where there are bone metastases, e.g. from breast, lung, prostate or thyroid primaries. Prednisolone enteric-coated 20 mg daily after a first injection of 100 mg hydrocortisone; phosphorus (Phosphate-Sandoz) one tablet three times a day; mithramycin 25 μg per kg of body weight – two injections at an interval of 24 hours.

Vomiting from cerebral causes Dexamethasone 4 mg four times a day as tablets or injection. After two weeks gradually reduce the dose to 2–4 mg daily. This treatment reduces tumour oedema but the improvement may only last for a few weeks (occasionally for several months in slow-growing tumours) as the tumour itself continues to grow. Symptom remission resulting from dexamethasone is only temporary and when the symptoms return there is little purpose in continuing the dexamethasone.

Intestinal obstruction This is usually impossible to relieve in terminal illness by surgery although this may be considered in appropriate cases, for instance if it is thought that the patient may have several months to live.

Pain and nausea are treated by analgesic and anti-emetic drugs which may be given per rectum or by injection. If injections are needed regularly the drugs may be given via a Greaseby Syringe Driver. The patient may continue to vomit once or twice a day but the pain and constant nausea can be relieved by appropriate medication.

Hyoscine 0.4 mg by injection is useful for both pain and vomiting of intestinal obstruction.

Naso-gastric tubes and intravenous fluid are nearly always unnecessary but it is important to maintain mouth care and moisturization of mucous membranes.

Fear and anxiety   Sometimes emotional tension could be a cause of nausea and vomiting. If the patient is obviously fearful or anxious, helping him to talk about his fears and worries may relieve the situation. Anxiolytic drugs may be prescribed, such as diazepam 2–5 mg three times a day – also as syrup, injections or suppositories 5 mg or 10 mg; lorazepam 1 mg twice a day – also as 2.5 mg tablet or 4 mg injection. Depression may be helped by mianserin 30–60 mg at night.

Even when the vomiting is controlled, the dying patient may worry that the symptom could return, and needs the assurance that a receptacle and tissues are near at hand although discreetly out of sight.

Meticulous care of the mouth is of course important, and changing of clothes and bed-linen if soiled so that the patient and his family do not suffer the additional distress of unpleasant odour. Another problem that the nurse must assist with is the accompanying anorexia and disinclination to take ordinary amounts of fluid. Suggested measures to ameliorate the situation are discussed later in this chapter.

Problems with bladder and bowels

Healthy adults take for granted the smooth functioning of their excretory system, particularly that of disposal of urine and faeces. In Western society these are very private matters performed to a greater or lesser degree without onlookers. When something becomes seriously wrong with an individual's excretory system it understandably is the cause of much worry and psychological threat, quite apart from physical symptoms. In caring for dying patients, the nurse will meet a number of common problems, and must be prepared to deal with them.

Problems of the urinary tract can cause great distress to a dying patient, particularly incontinence and urinary infection. Urinary retention and frequency of micturition can both be due to intrapelvic tumours affecting the bladder.

Incontinence of urine
The patient may be incontinent because of drugs, e.g. diuretics; infection; neurological problems; urinary fistula; anxiety.

Giving nursing care

Aims of care

1   To be prepared to catheterize any patient with severe frequency or incontinence in order to maintain comfort.

2   To pay particular attention to hygiene of the genital area.

3   To preserve the patient's independence in using the lavatory or commode for as long as possible.

4   To administer any drugs prescribed by the doctor to alleviate symptoms.

5   To ensure that the patient drinks sufficient fluids for as long as he is able to do so.

There should be no hesitation in catheterizing a patient who is in the terminal stage of an illness where incontinence is a problem. Alternatively a uridom may be used in the case of a man, and sometimes women patients will find the St Peter's Boat or Suba-seal urinal helpful. For some patients a paraplegic cushion with a space for a urinal may be the answer. When catheterization is chosen, an indwelling catheter should be inserted with 5–30 ml of water in the balloon. The cheap latex type of catheter may be used, although the more expensive silastic catheter is preferable being long lasting and not irritating to the mucous membrane. There is the advantage that the patient may only have to be subjected to one or two catheterizations throughout his last illness with the latter type of catheter. There is usually no problem with drainage even when the patient's fluid intake is below average. Bladder washouts are not often required but may be helpful should there be problems with drainage.

Care should also be given to the choice of drainage bag. Small, discreet leg bags are preferred by some with or without a drainage bag at night. Others will use the larger drainage bag but have it covered by clothing. Plastic 'driblet' bags are available and suitable for some men as an alternative to catheterization or other appliances. Both men and women patients can make use of Kanga pants and pads and these are available for all National Health Service patients. The Maxi-plus pants and pads (supplied by Molnlyck) are particularly comfortable and effective. The physiotherapist may be asked to help some patients by teaching them how to carry out pelvic floor exercises to improve control over micturition.

For all patients in their terminal illness it is most important that the nurse does everything possible to maintain continence. Assisting patients to the lavatory for as long as possible, or ensuring that a commode is within easy reach are important factors. Seat heights can be adjusted, or rails fixed beside the commode or in the toilet can help to maintain a degree of independence until the end. When bedpans and urinals are necessary these should be readily available and as comfortable as possible for the patient.

Urinary infections

These occur frequently in dying patients and the nurse may be the first to observe the onset, remembering that the signs and symptoms may appear unrelated to the urinary tract, for instance rigor, headache. An appropriate antibiotic is usually prescribed to relieve the painful and distressing symptoms often accompanying a urinary infection. If painful urethral spasm is present this may be relieved by one of the following drugs: flavoxate 200 mg three times a day; or phenazopyridine 200 mg three times a day.

Retention of urine

Retention of urine in the dying patient may be due to a number of causes, in particular infiltration of the urinary tract by malignant tumours or impacted faeces due to unrelieved constipation. It is usually necessary to pass a catheter but in the case of severe constipation, relief of this may solve the problem without resort to catheterization.

Constipation

Again, this symptom is very common in the terminal stage of most illnesses. The patient or relatives may mention the difficulty to the nurse, and rectal examination by the doctor may reveal a state of impacted faeces leading to a distressing and undignified situation for the patient.

Causes of constipation in the dying patient are the inevitable result of weakness and inactivity, diminished intake of food and fluid, and side effects of drugs especially opiates. A spurious diarrhoea sometimes accompanies severe constipation, and resolves when the hard faeces are removed. There may be a mechanical bowel obstruction caused, for example, by a malignant growth.

Giving nursing care

Aims of care

1   To deal with the present condition by clearing the rectum and lower bowel.

2   To take appropriate measures to prevent recurrence of constipation, which can include regular administration of aperients and rectal suppositories or enemas.

3   To show understanding of embarrassment and distress which the patient may feel, and afford privacy and ready availability of help with commode, bedpan or assistance to the lavatory as appropriate.

4   To attend to necessary hygiene.

The nurse must be constantly alert to the need for assisting the sluggish bowel to act and not relying on the patient's initiative in reporting difficulties. Regular aperients are needed for any patient having opiate drugs. These may take the form of bowel stimulants, for instance danthron (Dorbanex forte) syrup or capsules, or senna (Senokot) tablets. It is sometimes helpful to give a faecal softener, such as dioctyl sodium sulphosuccinate (Dioctyl forte). Bulk stimulants such as methylcellulose (Collogel) are less frequently used as it is often difficult to persuade the dying patient to take copious fluids, although it does help if as much fluid as possible is taken, especially fresh fruit drinks. While the patient is still able to take a fairly normal diet the addition of bran to selected items of food is useful.

Treatment of severe constipation

This must be relieved as soon as possible. The use of bisacodyl (Dulcolax) rectal suppositories may be successful but a phosphate enema is often required, given through a long rectal tube. An olive oil enema will be necessary where faeces are very hard; this should be retained for two hours if possible then followed by a phosphate enema. Sometimes a manual removal of faeces is the only possible course and a local anaesthetic lubricant such as lignocaine (Xylocaine) gel should be used to minimize discomfort. It may be necessary for the doctor to administer intravenous diazepam (Valium) to relax the anal sphincter before the procedure can be carried out without causing severe pain to the patient.

Diarrhoea

Unless there is some specific pathological reason, true faecal incontinence is uncommon in the dying patient until the last hours except where diarrhoea is present and the patient is unable to control this because of his weak state.

Causes of diarrhoea may be: certain drugs such as some antibiotics; radiotherapy; pancreatic tumours; tumours of the large intestine; bowel infection; anxiety and nervous tension.

Giving nursing care

Aims of care

1   To give appropriate treatment that will control the diarrhoea.

2   To carry out the necessary hygienic measures.

3   To preserve the patient's dignity.

Caring for a weak and ill patient suffering from diarrhoea requires sensitive and skilful nursing. Should the cause of the diarrhoea be due to constipation, the necessary suppositories, enemas or bowel washouts should be promptly given. Drugs prescribed by the doctor may include codeine phosphate 15 mg three times a day or diphenoxylate hydrochloride 2.5 mg and atropine sulphate 0.025 mg; these drugs have an opiate-like action and are usually effective. It is important to ensure that the patient discontinues this treatment as soon as the diarrhoea eases, so that subsequent constipation is avoided. Loperamide hydrochloride 2 mg in a dose of two capsules three times daily inhibits peristalsis. Steroid retention enemas – prednisolone (Predsol or Predenema) – are useful for persistent diarrhoea caused by radiotherapy or tumour infiltration; the pancreatin preparation Pancrex V is valuable as capsules or tablets given with food for steatorrhoea in this case. The use of a deodorant in the room would also be appreciated by the patient and family.

When present, anxiety and frustration should be recognized and careful counselling given by the appropriate person. Sometimes mild tranquillizers may be necessary, as diazepam 2–5 mg three times a day or lorazepam 1 mg twice a day.

While the diarrhoea still persists the nurse should ensure that the patient has easy access to a toilet or commode. Bedpans, if required, should be given promptly and courteously. A barrier cream should be applied to prevent chafing of the skin in the anal region. Where appropriate a supply of incontinence pants and pads should be given. Disposable sheeting can be used and save the patient the embarrassment of knowing that soiled sheets have to be laundered.

Diarrhoea is less common than constipation in the terminally ill patient, but is a distressing symptom.

Stomata

Care of a patient with colostomy or other stoma will depend largely on how long the patient has had it and his ability to cope with it (or the ability of a member of his family who has been used to helping in the matter). A patient with a long-established stoma will have become used to a particular type of appliance and his own way of dealing with this, and it is best to continue in the same way during the terminal illness. Obviously as the patient becomes weaker he may need help from nursing staff or family. Offering assistance as a patient loses control is always a sensitive step. Having a stoma is for many people a private affair and such matters as disposal of equipment may have been dealt with in a secret way, so the nurse needs to consider the patient's sensitivity here. She should also consult the patient as to his preferences in attending to the hygiene of the stoma. A nurse may have access to a nurse specialist, i.e. a stoma care nurse, if advice is needed.

Problems of abnormal stool, consistency, soreness of surrounding mucosa and skin or malignant tissue in the actual stoma or surrounding area may be present. The many firms specializing in stoma care equipment are always pleased to help with information about types of equipment.

Problems of nutrition and fluid intake

As the dying patient becomes increasingly unable to take a normal diet and variety and volume of fluids, the nurse must recognize that this fact in itself often causes great anxiety to the patient and also his family, due to the quite logical association with progressive weakness which is apparent to all.

There are several aspects to this problem, which are as follows:

1   There may be an obstructive lesion in the gastrointestinal tract (or upper respiratory tract) preventing the normal ingestion and passage of food and liquids. In the early stage of his disease, the patient with

such a problem may have commenced artificial feeding by nasogastric tube or gastrostomy tube.

2   Anorexia eventually becomes a problem for all dying patients no matter what the particular disease. There may be some underlying factors contributing to the lack of appetite, for instance certain types of therapy, e.g. cytotoxic drugs; nausea; constipation; gastrointestinal lesions; jaundice; uraemia; anxiety or depression; sore, dry or infected mouth; inappropriate diet offered.

During the last 48 hours of life, the patient becomes increasingly unable to take any nourishment by mouth, and only sips of fluids, before lapsing into unconsciousness.

Helping the patient to eat and drink
In everyday life the average person in reasonable health enjoys his meals and 'feels better' for them. There are psychological as well as physical reasons for this. Likewise, the patient who is terminally ill benefits from a balanced intake of food and fluids in the form of ordinary meals for as long as possible, even though the helpings of food will usually be small. The reasons for encouraging the patient to eat and drink are as follows:

1   Taking regular fluids, if necessary as small, frequent drinks, will help to keep the mouth moist and fresh and thus more comfortable. Fungal and other oral infections are common in the dying patient, and some of the drugs in common use cause dryness of the mouth. Together with oral hygiene, frequent drinks will help to lessen the discomfort of these conditions. It will also prevent concentration of urine and lessen the risk of urinary infection.

2   Eating a certain amount of solid food, containing some roughage, helps to counteract constipation, and again, chewing of this food encourages salivation and a moist mouth. The risk of pressure sores with their attendant pain and discomfort is ever-present in the dying patient. Regular intake of protein helps to prevent this, in whatever food the patient can best assimilate it.

3   While the patient remains alert, every effort should be made for his life to be as normal and pleasurable as possible. This includes making it possible for the continuation of enjoyment in eating and drinking especially in the company of others. As a result of this, the patient's

family will also gain comfort; one of the problems which causes a feeling of helplessness and misery especially for wives and mothers is an inability to carry out their usual role of sustaining their husband or child at mealtimes.

Helping to maintain appetite
Aims of care

1 Involving the patient and relatives in choosing an appropriate diet.

2 Flexibility of approach with regard to times of meals.

3 Carrying out any prescribed medical treatment which may improve the patient's appetite, or any nursing measures to alleviate a contributory cause of anorexia.

The first consideration is to control any distressing symptoms which are preventing the patient from wanting to eat or drink. Pain control is important from this point of view, and above all, the relief of nausea and vomiting. Control of all these symptoms has already been discussed in detail. It should be remembered that it sometimes takes a little while for an anti-emetic drug to take effect, and that it may be necessary to try more than one drug for the most effective result, or even give a combination of two drugs. A sore, unpleasant-tasting mouth will also be a deterrent to the desire to eat.

The administration of small doses of steroids, for example, will usually have a stimulating effect on the appetite and the effect is appreciated by patients especially if they have previously experienced a period of anorexia. Once their appetite has returned to some extent, many patients long for a particular dish which they enjoyed in the past. One lady suddenly requested and enjoyed on several days in September a consignment of mince pies because they had always given her pleasure at Christmas!

It should be mentioned that patients who have been taking relatively large doses of steroid drugs for a specific medical reason can develop an abnormal appetite during their terminal illness with constant craving for food. This can be distressing and embarrassing for the patient and present a dilemma for the doctor.

Small amounts of alcohol are often enjoyed, as an aperitif such as sherry, or taken with a meal, especially if the patient has been used to this in the past.

Presenting food and drink   Once the patient's appetite has been restored, he will often enjoy small helpings of food at normal meal times to within a day or two of his death.

This is more likely to happen if the patient's particular likes and dislikes can be studied, and the food attractively presented. Relatives will appreciate being invited to help here, and flexibility should be allowed for favourite tit-bits to be brought in. Too strict an adherence to previous diets for medical reasons is out of place at this stage. Care should be taken to avoid nausea. It has been noted that sweet foods are more likely to cause this than savoury ones.

There will be some patients who have special needs for cultural or religious reasons. They will be grateful for any efforts that can be made to find food to their liking. Most patients like small pieces of fresh fruit if prepared in an easy way for them to handle and eat, and this also helps in moistening the mouth. Patients should not be hurried; the weak individual will naturally be slow in eating.

Gradually the dying patient will only tolerate minimal amounts of food, and it will be a challenge to the nurse to give fluids which will both hydrate and nourish the patient as far as is possible. There are a number of well-known high-protein supplements such as Complan or Build-up which can be used. Egg flips can be offered, although not all patients like these. Virtually any drink that the patient will take should be available. The savoury tang of Bovril or Marmite drinks may be enjoyed, although their saltiness may not be acceptable if the patient tends to have a sore mouth or lips. Fizzy drinks are often useful; if too gaseous they can be diluted with water. The older patient may not be so keen on cold drinks, and prefer the well-loved cup of tea.

Helping patients to take their drink will be an important part of nursing care; the dying patient will eventually become too weak to hold the cup or glass himself and thus need the help of the nurse or a member of the family. Drinks should be provided willingly at any time of the day or night at the patient's request, and also given at frequent, regular intervals when the patient is unable to ask for them.

Patients suffering from dry mouths because of certain drugs can benefit from having methylcellulose solution with an appropriate flavour added to sip between meals, while they are still able to eat.

While the aim will be to encourage a fluid intake of about 1 litre in 24 hours for as long as possible, gradually the patient will not manage this and in a slowly deteriorating terminal illness will eventually only take sips of fluid, and small ice chips, before lapsing into unconsciousness. There may be some fundamental problem at the beginning of the terminal stage of an illness which makes eating and drinking difficult or impossible. The decision as to whether it is ethically right to institute some form of artificial feeding for certain patients is discussed in Chapter 16.

CHAPTER 4

NURSING AIMS AND GIVING CARE II
SISTER HELENA McGILLY, BERYL MUNNS
and JOY ROBBINS

PROBLEMS INVOLVING THE SKIN AND MUCOUS MEMBRANE   Sister Helena McGilly

The skin, being such a vital organ, will reflect many aspects of the dying patient's bodily and mental state and may be the cause of discomfort if not actual suffering. In assessing the condition of the skin the nurse may have observed abnormalities of *colour* – of the face and sometimes over the whole body:

Pallor – possibly due to anaemia, or apprehension.

Jaundice – due to disease of the liver or biliary tract.

Cyanosis – due to cardiac or respiratory disease.

Cachexia – the typical greyish facial hue with gaunt cheeks commonly seen in patients with advanced cancer, and accompanying other symptoms.

Petechiae – scattered bleeding of small blood vessels – abnormalities common in renal failure and blood dyscrasias.

and of *texture*:

Dryness – due to dehydration.

Sweating – may be due to fever and fear.

Shiny, taut skin with underlying swelling – oedema.

The puffy, moon-face (Cushing's syndrome) may accompany steroid drug therapy.

Pressure sores – these can occur in the terminal stage of any disease and range from small abrasions to deep cavities.

Widespread scratch marks – the patient's reaction to intense itching which causes much misery. The underlying cause may be obstructive jaundice, or allergic reaction to drug therapy.

Pressure sores   Any patient in the terminal stage of an illness is at risk with regard to developing pressure sores, irrespective of the particular disease, as the body systems deteriorate, especially the vascular system. With an inefficient blood supply and diminished metabolic activity in the tissues it is not surprising that sores develop easily. There may be other factors contributing to the risk, such as emaciation or the presence of gross sacral and ankle oedema. Increasing weakness means that the patient is less able to turn himself in bed or to shift his position if sitting in a chair. Once the first signs of an incipient pressure sore appear – i.e. an unhealthy redness of the skin – tissue break-down can proceed at an alarming rate until the distressing situation develops of a large necrotic area which becomes infected and causes sloughing to take place.

Fungating lesions   These are most common in breast cancer, but may occur in many other sites, such as lymph node metastes in neck or axilla. They may also occur in mucous membranes such as are in the vagina or rectum.

Bodily orifices   As all systems of the body begin to deteriorate, the dying patient becomes particularly vulnerable to inflammation and infection of the mouth, and sometimes of eyes and nostrils. In some circumstances, fistulae may occur between different sites, for instance rectum and vagina. This will result in inflammation and ulceration of mucosa exacerbated by excretions passing over the surface of the vagina. All of these problems are likely to cause much discomfort and pain to the patient.

Stomata   The patient may have an artificial opening onto the skin as a direct result of his present disease process, particularly in malignant disease, or incidental to this. Colostomy and ileostomy are common; gastrostomy may also be present. These may be well managed, or present problems of inflammation of skin and mucous membrane.

Giving nursing care

Aims of care

1   To give meticulous care to the cleanliness of the skin.
2   To try to prevent pressure sores by relieving pressure on vulnerable areas, and protecting the skin.
3   To relieve the pain and discomfort of lesions of the skin and mucous membranes by appropriate topical treatment and administration of other drugs, e.g. by oral route.
4   If there is a problem of odour, to take steps to minimize this.

Care of the skin, and general toilet   Washing the patient's skin should be carried out with due regard for personal preferences. Being immersed in a warm bath can be very relaxing and soothing, and even a very ill patient can find this procedure pleasurable. On the other hand there should not be a relentless routine approach either to giving the patient a bath in bed or in the bathroom. Timing is important so that the patient does not feel exhausted. If an over-all wash cannot be tolerated at a particular time, washing the face with special care of the eyes, the axillae and groins will meet the need to make the patient feel fresh and comfortable.

The patient should be allowed to do as much for himself as he wishes, the nurse helping with areas of difficulty such as the feet and back, and assisting with manicure of finger and toe-nails. Women patients will appreciate interest in using their favourite brand of talcum powder and perfume. Care of the hair is vital in both sexes for comfort and appearance; this is something which a relative who wishes to help can be asked to do if the patient cannot manage. A visit from the hairdresser when appropriate can be a great morale booster. Men should be helped to shave daily for the same reason.

Prevention of pressure sores   First, the patient should be encouraged to be out of bed for as much of the day as he feels able; this activity will, of course, gradually come to an end. Once the patient needs to be in bed all the time, regular turning and attention to all pressure areas must be carried out meticulously, which will include maintaining cleanliness of the skin and using an appropriate barrier cream if considered helpful. As with other patients at special risk of developing pressure sores, a suitable aid should be used, such as sheep skin, ripple mattress or foam mattress. It should be remembered that the patient sitting in a chair needs to have regular change of position and a pressure-relieving aid no less than the patient in bed. The use of an indwelling catheter for the dying patient who is incontinent of urine will prevent maceration of the skin and lessen the risk of pressure sores developing.

Wounds   Sometimes the dying patient will have a wound varying from a healing post-operative one to a large ulcerated lesion which includes pressure sores. Patients with cancer may have external growths which require attention, the main cause being breast cancer. These will vary from a dry, undressed area to a large, discharging, open wound, ulcerated and with an offensive odour. This will require frequent cleansing, dressing and reassessing. A swab may be requested by the doctor and an appropriate antibiotic ordered. Various types of agent are used to clean the wound, such as eusol and liquid paraffin; chlorhexidine (Hibitane 1/1000); hydrogen peroxide; normal saline; savlon. Various types of dressing material can be used, such as the traditional gauze or gamgee, sometimes soaked in the lotion. Newer agents are Foam Elastomer or Varidase.

If the patient is in a hospital or hospice, he may ask to be cared for in a side-room off the ward, and this is understandable. Efforts should be made to lessen the isolation by treating the patient like any other – sitting close to him, and talking in a normal way with him. If sinuses or fistulae are present, they need to be well cleansed. The lotion of choice may be noxythiolin (Noxyflex), using a syringe or catheter to irrigate. If the drainage is profuse, a colostomy bag may be fitted. This will reduce the frequency of the dressings, prevent soiling of clothes and reduce odour.

Yoghurt is sometimes used as a dressing for a fungating lesion, being soothing and deodorizing in effect. Such a dressing will need to be changed at least once during 24 hours. If the patient is having antibiotics, this may defeat the result of the dressing because the antibiotics may destroy the lactobacillus. Gauze dressings impregnated with soft paraffin ointment (tulle gras) are helpful in preventing sticking of the dressing and therefore in reducing pain in the area.

Wounds which leak may be sealed in cellophane paper or a colostomy bag adapted to fit over the wound. This will also help to control the odour. For this purpose a deodorant such as Nilodor may be applied to the outer dressing, or charcoal pads used. This problem can be distressing to the patient and relatives and it is worth trying to find the most effective measure to diminish the odour. Occasionally patients may benefit from a surgical debridement of the wound, carried out in an operating theatre. Malignant growths which destroy the bony structure of the face present a challenge to the nurse not only in the physical care needed but because of the severe mental distress that the patient will often experience. While dealing with the dressing of the cavity the nurse should be careful to show no sign of repugnance. Irrigation is sometimes used by pouring normal saline through an infusion set and collecting the fluid.

Intense itching   If severe, this can cause great distress and misery to the dying patient, whose threshold of tolerance is likely to be low. The nurse will be asked to apply an appropriate topical application according to the cause of the irritation. Oral medication may also be prescribed. Fungal infections are common, especially in the inguinal and perianal regions, and pruritus often accompanies jaundice and uraemia.

Oedema   There may be many causes of generalized oedema in the terminally ill patient. Specific treatment is rarely given but the nurse may be asked to administer diuretic drugs if it is thought to be helpful.

Localized oedema may result in massive enlargement of a limb, especially of an arm in women patients following radical mastectomy. This is most uncomfortable, and the use of a Jobst pump may be effective. This is an inflatable cushion which is applied to the limb, completely surrounding it. The cushion is connected to a small, electrically driven motor, exerting continuous pressure for about 20 minutes, which disperses the excess fluid back into the circulation. This gives considerable relief although it does not prevent eventual recurrence of the oedema. The same treatment can be used for oedema of the legs. Any other means to make the patient more comfortable, such as the judicious use of cushions or footstools to support limbs, should be tried.

The nurse may be asked to assist the doctor in removing ascitic fluid in a dying patient if this is causing distress because of distension or breathlessness. The patient is catheterized and when the abdomen is tapped the fluid will be allowed to drain away slowly. Injection of Coparvax (*Corynebacterium parvum*: Wellcome) 7 mg ampoule diluted and injected into the peritoneal cavity after draining away the fluid is effective in preventing recurrence in about 60% of cases.

MOUTH CARE IN TERMINAL ILLNESS
Beryl Munns

Good mouth care is important in all areas of nursing and in addition there are extra factors that demand close observation and attention when patients are dying. This section briefly discusses two main subject areas:

1   The reasons why mouth care may be of special importance in terminal illness.
2   The components of mouth care for such patients.

Mouth deterioration is not inevitable in the dying patient. Perhaps this is the most important reason for giving the correct care, since mouths may then be kept in a good condition. It has been noted that they may be restored even in the face of rapid general deterioration.

Problems involving the mouth
Poor mouths have bad physical and psychological effects. A dry mouth will often feel unpleasant and result in difficulty with eating. One dying patient with candidiasis described the feeling as: 'If I put my tongue in fizzy lemonade it would go zzzzzzzzzz.' When a patient knows that his mouth is not quite right there is fear of halitosis and consequent withdrawal from others. All these situations diminish the quality of life. Terminally ill patients are often elderly and have denture problems. If there has been loss of weight these do not fit properly and rubbing may produce open sores which may proceed to infection because the wearing of dentures occludes air from oral surfaces. Patients may have been deteriorating over a long period during which weakness has reduced their ability to care for their mouths. In his last days a patient may lack full consciousness and the ability to complain of a distressing mouth condition. He may also be unable to experience the sensation that would

---

*The author gratefully acknowledges the help of the Elizabeth Clark Trust.

warn of trouble. Other reasons why mouth care is especially important in dying patients are:

1   Terminally ill patients have often had inadequate diets for long periods if they have been experiencing nausea and vomiting for some time or have been living alone and unable to make the effort to obtain a balanced diet. Other patients, for instance those having steroids, tend to assuage their hunger with excessive carbohydrate intake. Unless the debris is removed adequately there can be a very rapid deterioration of the gingiva, increasing greatly the patient's general misery.

2   Very sick patients are often reluctant to eat and drink. One of the effects is that the salivary glands are then not stimulated to function. This results in poor clearance of the mouth and debris left as a focus of infection.

3   Candidiasis is associated with various diseases; among these are malignant conditions, especially the leukaemias, infections and diabetes mellitus.

4   Many drugs affect the mouth including those given previously to many terminally ill patients. Examples are immunosuppressive agents, corticosteroids and antibiotics.

Giving nursing care
Aims of care

1   To prevent mouth deterioration by regular observation and choice of the most suitable cleansing agents.
2   To maintain a clean, comfortable mouth with the patient's co-operation.
3   To report any abnormality immediately so that appropriate treatment may be instituted without delay.

Regular observation of the whole mouth   This should be daily for patients whose condition is weak and deteriorating. It is often a practice to observe the tongue alone but candidal infection and other disorders can affect all the oral mucosae. The most natural and least disturbing time for this inspection is when the patient would normally be receiving mouth care and removing dentures. Many patients are so weak or suffer such nausea that it is a real effort for them to take out a denture, particularly if it is a close-fitting one. Any deviation from the normal appearance of the tissues should be promptly reported to medical staff.

Encouragement towards self-help Whenever possible, mouth care is best undertaken by the patient, with assistance if necessary to provide help and confidence. The patient alone will know the tender spots and those where pressure would cause retching. Those who have difficulty swallowing or breathing may find mouth care a very frightening procedure. If in an unhurried way they can be gently helped to control the process then confidence will be gained.

Care tailored to the needs of the individual This includes both the timing and the process of care. It may be sufficient for ambulant patients with reasonable appetites to clean and refresh their mouths after meals; the unconscious patient, particularly the mouth breather will require 2-hourly attention. This should be given when he is lying on his side, great care being taken that he does not aspirate any fluid. Other patients who have dry mouths and anorexia have been found to benefit from oral care before meals so that salivary glands and appetite are stimulated.

The agents of care There are many different traditions of care which have been derived through the experience of years rather than any systematic and scientific investigation. Research findings will be quoted in this section and they indicate a need for further enquiry. Some research suggests that the process rather than the agent of care is the important factor.

Removing debris A soft small toothbrush combined with unwaxed dental floss is found to be most effective for removing debris from all surfaces of the teeth. The electric rotating type of toothbrush was found excellent in one study, for use by patient or nurse. Access to all areas was made easier. Toothbrush heads were kept in 1% sodium hypochlorite solution. Foam sticks and a swabbed finger have been found to be the next most acceptable tools by nurse and patient, although more effective for removing debris from the soft tissues than from the teeth. Mouthwashes only remove loose debris.

An effervescent action is necessary to remove mucus and crusts and both sodium bicarbonate (one half teaspoon to 1 pint water) and hydrogen peroxide 3% (diluted 1:4) are used as mouthwashes. It is, however, suggested that these preparations are only used when strictly necessary as both have potential to damage the oral mucosa and sodium bicarbonate has an unpleasant taste. As a more pleasant provider of mechanical action half a vitamin C tablet may be dissolved on the tongue.

One small piece of research indicated that a mixture of mouthwash, ice chips and tap water applied to the tissues might reduce the surface tension and penetrate the mucous barrier, stimulate the blood flow and, through friction, remove the remaining sordes which could then be rinsed out with the mixture.

Moistening, softening, freshening, stimulating Mouthwashes moisten and soften the tissues although their refreshing effect is thought to be very transient. Mild commercial mouthwashes may be used or normal saline. Redoxan mouthwashes have been found to be useful when patients have a fear of swallowing other types. Research indicates that chlorhexidine (Corsodyl) has an anti-plaque effect.

Fruit juices also play a part in the care of the mouth, where they moisten, refresh and stimulate. Pineapple chunks may be chewed, grapefruit juice may be sipped and lemon juice, often combined with glycerine, applied to tissues. Lemon stimulates the salivary glands but caution has to be taken over the frequency of application otherwise there may be a 'reflex exhaustion' effect. Chewing gum, preferably the non-sugar type, may also help in the stimulation of salivary glands. When the mouth remains very dry there are various forms of artificial saliva that may be sipped or applied to the mouth surfaces.

Caring for the lips This is an important area, for dryness can soon develop in very painful cracks that provide sites for candidal infection. Lips may be cleansed gently with saline swabs and KY jelly, vaseline or glycerine applied. Care needs to be taken with the latter two as they are thought to be potentially harmful if aspirated.

Fluid and diet control There is controversy at present over the relation of general hydration to moisture in the mouth but one researcher concluded that the patient who was reluctant to eat and drink was more at risk of dehydration and poor condition than the patient having tube feeds or intravenous fluids. When there is a mouth problem high-moisture foods should be encouraged as well as the maximum amount of fluids that the patient can drink. Diet control that is consistent with keeping the patient happy can be attempted with the patient who feels constantly hungry. Less sweet items may be offered between meals or perhaps the eating of sticky items can be timed shortly before mouth care is due.

Reporting abnormalities   All abnormalities should be reported as soon as possible, for not only does the smallest lesion create disproportionate discomfort but when the patient is very debilitated it is easy for candidal infections to take a rapid hold. A variety of antifungals may be prescribed using either a local or systemic approach. In the case of local applications it is important that the suspension or contents of a medicated lozenge be allowed to come in contact with all the oral surfaces. This will not be the case if the patient is wearing dentures. The patient should hold the suspension for as long as possible before swallowing, and twice daily when dentures are cleaned, they should be coated with antifungal. It is important to note any directions that relate to the treatment, for example sodium bicarbonate should not be used when the patient is receiving nystatin (Nystan), as it is thereby rendered less effective. Finally patients should always be encouraged to complete the prescribed course to help prevent recurrence.

References

Bruya M, Madeira and Powell, N (1966) Effects of agents used for oral hygiene, American Journal of Nursing, 75: 1349–1352

Daeffer R (1980) Oral hygiene measures for patients with cancer I, Cancer Nursing, 3 (5), Oct: 347–356

Daeffler R (1980) Oral hygiene measures for patients with cancer II, Cancer Nursing, 3 (6), Dec: 427–432

Daeffler R (1981) Oral hygiene measures for patients with cancer III, Cancer Nursing, 4 (1), Feb: 29–35

Ginsberg, M K (1961) A study of oral hygiene nursing care, American Journal of Nursing, 61: 67–69

Harris, M D (1980) Tools for mouth care, Nursing Times, Feb 21: 340–342

Hilton, D (1980) Oral hygiene and infection, Nursing Times, July 17: 1270–1280

Howarth, H (1977) Mouth care procedures for the very ill, Nursing Times, March 10: 354–355

Kirkis, E J (1978) This oral care technique gets results, RN Magazine, 41 (10), Oct: 82

Passos, J Y and Brand, L M (1966) Effects of agents used for oral hygiene, Nursing Research, 15: 196–202

Sharon, A et al. (1977) The effect of chlorhexidine mouth rinses on oral candida in a group of leukaemic patients, Oral Surgery, 44: 201–205

Shepherd, J P (1978) The management of the oral complication of leukaemia, Oral Surgery, 45: 543–548

Wallace, J and Freeman, P A (1978) Mouth care in patients with blood dyscrasias, Nursing Times, June 1: 921–922

RESPIRATORY PROBLEMS   Joy Robbins

There are a number of diseases in which symptoms related to the respiratory tract may become very distressing to the patient during the terminal stage of the illness. The commonest symptoms are: cough; excessive, sometimes purulent or blood-stained sputum; dyspnoea; haemoptysis; chest pain.

Causes of dyspnoea in a dying patient may be the result of a chronic condition such as asthma, chronic bronchitis or congestive cardiac failure, or of a malignant tumour infiltrating the lungs and other parts of the respiratory tract.

Pneumonia is common in the terminal stage of many illnesses. Fear or anxiety may produce dyspnoea which itself leads to further tension and thus a vicious circle of cause and effect. Cough is another problem which may be present in association with dyspnoea, and sometimes from the same cause.

Giving nursing care
Aims of care

1   To provide the most comfortable physical position to ease the patient's dyspnoea or cough.
2   To administer drugs and assist with other forms of treatment prescribed by the doctor.
3   To co-operate with the physiotherapist if required.
4   To try to lessen emotional tension which may be aggravating the dyspnoea.

General principles of care
Positioning the patient   Most patients with respiratory problems are

more comfortable when sitting upright. They will need plenty of pillows, and some form of back-rest. Some patients are more at ease sitting in an armchair, than in bed, and may insist on doing so for much of the time until they lose consciousness.

When towards the end a patient is almost comatose, a distressing symptom may occur which is commonly known as the 'death rattle'. This is mainly due to secretions present in the trachea which the patient is too weak to cough up. Although it is unlikely that the patient is troubled by this, it is unpleasant for relatives and other patients to hear, if the patient is in an open ward. The patient should be placed on his side in a semi-prone position with head low, and the doctor will usually prescribe an injection of atropine or hyoscine to suppress the secretions.

Mouth care   The nurse should remember that respiratory symptoms are often accompanied by a dry and unpleasant-tasting mouth, so mouth care becomes even more important.

Fear and anxiety   Some respiratory symptoms arouse great fear and anxiety in the patient, which have repercussions on the family. The patient with dyspnoea may feel that he is suffocating and the panic induced will increase the dyspnoea, thus a vicious circle is set up. Haemoptysis is frightening and unpleasant, and the patient may have several episodes and a final catastrophic one occurring at the time of death. The nurse and the doctor together can do much to minimize this distress, by ensuring that the patient is never left alone, and by use of medication.

Special measures

Cough   This may be dry and unproductive, making the patient exhausted. Steam inhalations may be helpful, and the use of a linctus, such as methadone linctus 2 mg in 5 ml. Sips of hot drinks are soothing.

A productive cough with mucopurulent sputum may be relieved by a broad-spectrum antibiotic given for a few days, such as chloramphenicol 250 mg four times a day. The physiotherapist will be invaluable in helping with postural drainage and gentle chest percussion.

Dyspnoea   This symptom often frightens the patient, and the relatives too, and, as pointed out, becomes worse with fear and anxiety. The nurse should make sure that the patient is not left alone, and that a subdued light is by the bed at night.

When the patient feels particularly distressed, having him facing an open window and feeling the air on his face can be comforting. In some cases, administration of oxygen for short periods may be tried although the benefit is likely to be psychological rather than physical; sitting with the patient and listening to his fears should accompany these efforts.

Drugs will be prescribed according to the cause of dyspnoea, for instance diuretics in the case of pulmonary oedema, and if the patient is already having an opiate drug regularly for pain control this will help to reduce the rate of breathing. A treatment which can be quite effective in some patients is the inhalation of a local anaesthetic, such as bupivacaine hydrochloride (Marcain) 0.5% via a Bird Nebulizer or Palmosonic inhaler. This treatment anaesthetizes the lung receptors which are situated in the alveoli and also other receptors in the bronchioles and trachea. The result is a reduction of the subjective sensation of breathlessness. This is also very useful for the chronic unproductive cough which occurs in tracheolaryngitis. Finally, anxiolytic drugs will be prescribed; sometimes a dramatic improvement may be obtained by an injection of diazepam (Valium) where the emotional overlay is high.

Haemoptysis The patient may have had several small warning haemorrhages, and if in hospital or hospice, it will be advisable to have him in a single room if a final massive haemoptysis is anticipated. Red towels should be available to protect the bed, the idea being to minimize the distressing effect for the patient. A suction machine should also be at hand. Immediately a massive haemorrhage occurs, the doctor should be summoned and will give the patient an appropriate dose of an opiate drug by injection, taking into account what the patient is already receiving. Further active treatment such as blood transfusion is not now appropriate and the patient will lose consciousness and die peacefully. A member of the family may wish to sit by the bed and hold the patient's hand during this time, but a member of the staff should be present as well.

This is a difficult experience for the nurse and doctor when in other circumstances the instinctive reaction is to take heroic measures, if necessary, to stop the bleeding and restore the patient to health as far as possible. The family, if present, will need particular support and assurance that the patient died without pain and further distress.

Tracheostomy It is not uncommon for the nurse to care for a terminally ill patient who has a tracheostomy, usually performed for a malignant condition. The actual care of the tracheostomy site will be the same as for any other patient, but the dying patient will need special understanding regarding his need for communication, as he becomes weaker. If he has been dealing with the tracheostomy himself he may feel anxious about having to leave this to a nurse whom he does not know when admitted to a hospital, if he is too weak to continue. Having one or two nurses only to deal with this will inspire confidence as they get to know the patient and his needs. There may be a member of the family who has become skilled in the matter and should be consulted about any detail of information that will be helpful; indeed, he or she should be allowed to continue to help with the procedure if desired.

PROBLEMS ASSOCIATED WITH LOCOMOTION
Joy Robbins

Many dying patients have few problems of this nature until the last few days of their illness, when increasing weakness overtakes them. Other patients may become virtually immobile for many weeks or months during the terminal stage of their illness. This may be as a direct result of neurological, cardiovascular or muscular disorders or as a signal to certain forms of malignant disease. Some patients may indeed have had years of immobility due to a chronic neurological disease, such as multiple sclerosis, so that the terminal stage is simply a continuation of the problem.

Dangers of immobility are similar at any stage of an illness, notably: pressure sores; pneumonia; muscle wasting; joint contractures. Apart from these potential dangers, the patient who is unable to move without help will often become physically uncomfortable, and psychologically frustrated.

Giving nursing care
Aims of care

1   To organize a regular programme of changing the patient's position whether in bed or sitting in a chair.
2   To ensure that all limbs are gently exercised and placed in anatomically correct positions.

3   To avoid over-tiring the patient in any therapeutic endeavour.

4   To co-operate with the physiotherapist in her efforts for the patient's comfort.

The patient whose terminal illness is advancing rapidly may become frustrated and depressed at increasing weakness; sometimes considerable patience is needed to tolerate anger and irritation from the patient who has always had an independent and strong personality. Placing everything within easy reach when the patient can no longer walk is important, and appropriate physiotherapy will help to diminish the usual risks of immobility such as stiffness of joints and pressure sores.

The patient should be allowed and helped to move about to whatever extent he wishes. There is a moving story of a woman patient who was becoming physically weaker and obviously feeling very tired and lethargic. On certain mornings, when her husband was to visit in the afternoon, she replied to the nurse who enquired if she would like a bath: 'No, I shall just lie on the bed to save all my energy for this afternoon when my husband likes to take me out for a little outing round the garden in my wheelchair.' When the husband came, his visible satisfaction at giving his wife what he thought was an eagerly anticipated pleasure in her day, was very evident. This true story illustrates an important truth in relationships between dying people and those they love. Both husband and wife knew that time was short and yearned to share their love in the few tangible ways left to them. The wife died knowing that in hiding her own weakness and disinclination for physical effort she gave much pleasure to her husband. In his bereavement the husband found comfort in remembering the little service that he gave to his wife, thinking that it had 'made her day' on each occasion. Quite rightly, the nurse did not remonstrate or interfere with the wife's decision.

A patient with a malignant disease of the bone is liable to sustain one or more pathological fractures. If this occurs in the pre-terminal stage of the disease it is common for a surgical procedure to be carried out, usually some form of intramedullary pin and plating. During the terminal illness, further fractures may occur, presenting problems of immobility and difficulty in moving the patient without causing him excruciating pain. Further surgical intervention may be out of the question, and simple methods, such as applying skin traction or supporting the limb in a sling or on pillows, will be used.

In lifting the patient several people should help, and an unhurried gentle approach is essential. Before moving the patient, it is kind to consider whether an analgesic drug should be administered as a boost to the patient's regular pain control regimen. The advice and help of a physiotherapist will be valuable.

PSYCHOLOGICAL AND SPIRITUAL PROBLEMS
Joy Robbins

The nurse will meet many dying patients who exhibit anxiety or depression. It has already been noted that a sensitive approach and readiness to listen is important in assessing the patient's mood. *Causes* of anxiety and depression are multiple and may not become apparent at the first meeting with the nurse or doctor. The patient's confidence has first to be gained, and his right to reveal only as much of his inner thoughts as he wishes must be respected.

If he has some insight into his condition, a spiritual sadness may be present as he contemplates the ultimate mystery of death involving the loss of his own life, and parting from family and friends.

Understanding and meeting the psychological needs of patients has been woven into every chapter of this book since this aspect of a patient's care cannot be divorced from the physical component, nor from the attitudes and roles of the members of the caring team.

Emotional needs

The first priority is for the nurse to establish a relationship of trust with the patient. This will not develop if she gives an impression of wanting to hurry away on every occasion, and avoiding any real contact. By getting to know the patient she will have an awareness of his emotional state which of course can change from day to day. Personality, family attitudes, and his physical condition are among the factors which will influence emotions, and vice versa. The main emotional problems for which the patient needs help will now be discussed in outline, and developed in subsequent chapters.

Fear   A fear of how the final phase of dying will occur is common and may be linked with anticipation of certain intolerable physical events such as choking to death. If the patient can voice his fears to doctor and nurse, so that assurance can be given that these are unfounded, much relief will be given. Fear of the mystery of death and uncertainty as to an after-life may be helped by offering the services of a minister of religion, and is discussed in the section on spiritual care.

Loneliness   This is sometimes linked with fear if the patient feels there is no-one to whom he can turn to share the burden by listening to his problems. The nurse should be aware that the patient can still feel lonely in a ward full of other patients. Even if she is busy, a smile and pausing to enquire if the patient needs anything reinforces a sense of personal care. Providing companionship and suitable diversionary activity helps to dispel loneliness.

Anxiety   The patient may tend to be already of an anxious disposition and the facts of dying can produce many particular anxieties such as worries about finance and family well-being, and uncertainty about the prognosis of the illness. The nurse can play an important role in enlisting the help of other colleagues such as the social worker. To help the patient who becomes excessively anxious and agitated, drugs may be prescribed such as: diazepam 2–5 mg twice or three times a day; lorazepam 1 mg twice a day; clobazam 10 mg twice a day.

If a dying patient is receiving care in an institution he may express a great longing to see his own home again, and become restless and anxious. Even if the patient is weak, it may be justifiable to meet this request and arrange for him to be taken home for a short visit. It is found that the patient is often remarkably peaceful once he has achieved what he probably knows is a last farewell to his home.

Sadness   It is understandable that the dying patient who has insight into his condition experiences sadness at the impending loss of his life and all that he values, including those he loves. There is no easy remedy to prescribe for this natural reaction, but if the care given by all the caring team is of a high quality, the patient will at least be relieved of distressing symptoms which interfere with progress towards acceptance of his coming death. Where there are close family relationships, and both patient and family have reached acceptance together, the remaining span of life can take on a new and precious quality.

Depression   It is not always easy to distinguish sadness from depression, but important to treat the latter before it becomes severe and very distressing. The observations of the nurse will be vital, as the patient may assume a mask when the doctor visits, and the true state of affairs can be missed at first. A psychiatrist or clinical psychologist may be asked to see the patient, and antidepressant drugs will be prescribed. The timing is important, as these drugs do not usually have any significant effect until the patient has been taking them for about a week; this is a long time in terms of many terminal illnesses. An example of a useful anti-depressant drug with fewer side-effects than some is mianserin 20–30 mg taken at night.

Depression may be one cause of insomnia, although of course there are many others. The nurse will often be involved in trying to help a patient to sleep, first by investigating the possible causes. There can be a number of physical causes, or simple environmental problems such as noise or over-heating of the ward or room. Specific remedies should be tried first, including sitting with the patient and quietly discussing a possible solution with him. Eventually, some patients will need sedation, such as dichloralphenazone 650 mg or chlorpromazine 25–50 mg.

Confusion   The nurse may often have to care for a dying patient who is confused. This can occur from a number of causes: toxic – for instance, pneumonia; cerebral – especially tumours or metastases; biochemical – for instance, uraemia.

If the patient is elderly, admission to an institution from home may precipitate a mild senile dementia. The patient should be handled gently and calmly, and there should be no attempt to argue if he appears to be hallucinated. Sometimes a respiratory or urinary infection can cause confusion, and unless the patient is thought to be near death, treatment with appropriate antibiotics may produce a dramatic improvement.

It is not unknown for a dying patient to become confused due to alcohol withdrawal, and this will need skilled handling.

It is usually necessary to resort to medication if the patient is anxious as well as confused. Useful drugs are: diazepam 5–10 mg orally or by injection; chlormethiazole syrup 5–10 ml or capsules 1–2. This drug is especially useful for patients experiencing alcohol withdrawal.

Weakness and tiredness   One of the symptoms which will often result in the patient also feeling anxious or depressed is the lethargy and weakness associated with the gradual deterioration of the bodily systems. This is particularly noted in the state known as cachexia which is present in advanced cancer. The administration of corticosteroids – prednisolone (enteric-coated) 10 mg twice a day – is often useful in producing a subjective improvement in a feeling of well-being. If anaemia is the cause of the weakness, it may be appropriate to give a patient a blood transfusion. This symptom can be a trying one for the patient, but if all other symptoms are well-controlled it may not worry him unduly if the process is a gradual one.

Spiritual care

It is necessary to know exactly what is meant by 'spiritual care'. The immediate response might be – to help the patient to practise a religious faith in as far as he wishes. Many people, however, do not affirm any religious beliefs; have they therefore no need of spiritual care? This hinges on what is meant by 'spirit'. The Pocket Oxford Dictionary defines the word at some length, beginning thus:

Spirit   animating or vital principle of a person or animal. Intelligent or immaterial part of a person. Soul.

This further begs the question – what is meant by the soul?

Soul   spiritual or immaterial part of man regarded as immortal; moral, emotional or intellectual part of person or animal. A person, especially as embodying moral or intellectual qualities.

Finally, has this any link with psychological aspects? Yes, according to the same source:

Psyche   mind, soul.

This introduction is simply to show that the matter is somewhat complex. It would seem that spiritual and psychological matters cannot be separated into neat compartments. It can at least be agreed that the end of life is a time above all when the aims of the caring team are directed towards making the dying *person* as comfortable as possible – the spirit animating and holding together body, emotions and intellect. Therefore, spiritual care is an integral part of that service called 'total patient care'.

Religion provides a visible framework of support and guidance for human beings in their endeavour to lead a good life, and to prepare for the goal of a life hereafter. This rests on the belief in the immortality of the human spirit, and the help of a higher power than human beings, namely God. Death is seen as a gateway to an eternal life of perfect happiness. These spiritual beliefs, presented here in a simplistic way, have been of great solace to many dying people, although it is said that in Western society their numbers are declining. In Chapter 15 some details are given regarding the role of ministers of various religions in the spiritual care of patients and their families, and how the nurse can assist in bringing this service to her patients.

Many people will say that they believe in God and some kind of an after-life, without belonging to a particular religious faith. Others say that they believe that death is the end of the human person. Whatever her own attitudes, the nurse should ask such patients if there is anything that they would find helpful if they do not wish to have specific religious facilities. They may like to read, or have read to them, words from the world's great philosophers or religious leaders, including the Psalms or words from the Christian Gospels, or books of other world religions. In some hospices short prayers are said in the wards at the beginning and end of each day. Comments are often made by patients that they have found this custom a comfort to them. However, it would be intrusive to subject a patient to formal religious services in ward or chapel unless he wished to be present.

It should be remembered that in many religions certain physical actions and material objects used as symbols are very important to the believer, and should be respected. Some examples which the nurse may meet are described in Chapter 15.

Attitudes in giving care

Whenever the nurse is giving care to the dying patient, preservation of self-respect and dignity should be an integral part of the procedure. The older person is often exasperated by a body which has been taken for granted for many years and is now weak and unable to carry out activities previously performed in an automatic way to a greater or lesser degree. Such a patient may feel especially undermined by being attended by a nurse young enough to be a daughter or even granddaughter! A number of small but significant actions by the nurse can help to maintain the patient's self-respect and dignity as a human individual.

First, the patient is entitled to be called by the name and title that he chooses. Use of first names without permission can sound patronizing, and many older people will wish to be allowed the dignity of a title, for instance Miss, Mrs, Mr. In her turn, the nurse can put the patient at ease by telling him how she would like to be addressed. Where appropriate, patients should be consulted when decisions are to be made about their care. For instance, flexibility should be used in the timing of a patient's bath and not an insistence on its taking place when convenient for the nurse if the patient really does not feel like the procedure at that particular moment. In residential care, such matters as use of public television sets, accommodating those who wish to smoke, and conversely those who find proximity to a smoker uncomfortable, need sensitive handling by the nurse. Most patients respond to explanations of the needs of others when it is evident that the staff are doing their best for individual and collective needs.

When carrying out any physical care, lack of proper verbal preparation, addressing the patient as if he were an immature child, or indulging in too much superficial chatter can be distressing. This does not imply that a solemn face, whispered words or silence are needed. One learns by practice that a normal cheerful manner is supportive, and that the patient endowed with a sense of humour, and whose symptoms are well controlled, will enjoy joking with his nurses.

There are a number of procedures that patients may need to undergo which can be particularly disturbing to their sense of self-respect. Having one's teeth cleaned by another person, having the genital areas washed, and procedures involving insertion of substances into the rectum will be felt as acutely embarrassing and humiliating unless the nurse is sensitive and by her own approach demonstrates empathy with the patient's feelings.

Caring for the family

The important role of the family in helping to assess the patient's needs, by giving information on the admission of the patient to institution or home care programme has been described. The different members of the family will also have their own difficulties and needs which will vary according to circumstances and the environment in which the patient is receiving care, and these are discussed further in later chapters.

Relatives should be encouraged to help with the care of the dying member of the family in any way they wish. At home, they are the main carers; in an institution, they may not be able to give much physical care due to sheer tiredness from travel and coping with family responsibilities. They should be welcomed and praised for their demonstration of love by just being with the patient, and the time and effort it has taken to achieve this.

One common principle must always be acceptance that the family of whom the dying patient is a member have a right to be together as much as possible. The nurse will have a co-ordinating function here to facilitate this with other members of the team. For instance, the social worker may be asked to arrange financial assistance with fares for visiting purposes.

When meeting members of the family during the terminal illness of their relative and after the death, nurses sometimes feel ill at ease and inadequate in what they say. As with communication in the case of dying patients, it is attitudes and compassionate care being demonstrated that can be far more valuable than words. Being a good listener will be deeply appreciated. Enquiries as to how the family are coping, offers of help with transport and solicitude in offering cups of tea at the right moment speak of real interest and concern.

Evaluation of care

As a conclusion to these three chapters describing the process of nursing the dying patient it must be stressed that evaluation of the effectiveness of care should be frequent and regular. The patient's situation is often a constantly changing pattern and a swift response is needed to maintain comfort in the face of a new problem. Evaluation will involve listening to the patient's views and those of his family when making decisions. It requires that the nursing staff not only consult together to evaluate the care they are giving, but also meet with other colleagues to share their views, since all aspects of the needs of patient and family are inextricably linked.

References

Ainsworth-Smith, I and Speck, P (1982) Letting Go – Caring for the dying and bereaved, SPCK

Cockburn, M (1980) The dying patient and his family, in E Pearce (Editor) A General Textbook of Nursing, Faber and Faber

Downie, P A (1978) Cancer Rehabilitation – An introduction for physiotherapists and the allied professions, Faber and Faber

Hanratty, J F (1981) Control of Distressing Symptoms in the Dying Patient, St Joseph's Hospice

Hector, W and Whitfield, S (1982) Nursing Care for the Dying Patient and the Family, William Heinemann Medical Books

Krauss, M (1978) Terminal care, in R Tiffany (Editor) Cancer Nursing – Medical, Faber & Faber

Lamerton, R (1980) Care of the Dying, Pelican Books

Sampson, C (1982) The Neglected Ethic, McGraw-Hill

Saunders, C M (1978) The Management of Terminal Disease, Edward Arnold

CHAPTER 5

THE ROLE OF THE DOCTOR
JOHN COLLINS

The purpose of this chapter is to outline some of the special facets of the doctor's role in caring for dying patients. More details of practical management will be found in subsequent chapters; here the intention is to concentrate on the following: the doctor's approach; diagnosis; prognosis; patient and family. The treatment of specific symptoms or problems, will not be discussed in this chapter.

Viewpoint

The dying patient represents a peculiar problem for the modern doctor, whatever his speciality. Doctors today have a long, scientifically based general and professional education culminating in a degree of technical expertise hitherto unknown. This knowledge well befits them for solving the clinical problems of modern medical management of acutely ill patients.

Sadly though, in all this development something of the human face of medicine has been accidentally left by the wayside. Doctors so trained have a tendency to see their patients in terms of disease processes with known precipitants and consequences rather than as people with difficulties, often multiple, caused by or causing ill health.

The former approach is particularly unsuitable for some groups of patients, and must be seen to be so. It will not have escaped the notice of any health care worker today that technological medicine does not hold the whole answer for problems of, for instance, the pregnant mother, the unborn child, the handicapped child, the chronically sick, the mentally ill and the elderly.

The dying are one such group, and a very large one, including some 130 000 people dying each year in the United Kingdom from cancer.

It is the very unsuitability of modern medicine's management of this group's particular problems that has been the main stimulus to the development of alternative approaches to care for these patients. The hospice movement has fostered this alternative approach, studying and learning from dying patients in a scientific manner and applying the skills of doctors, nurses, social workers, physiotherapists and others to the 'total' care of dying patients. In so doing a wealth of knowledge has accumulated in all areas of terminal care. It is now never true that 'nothing can be done' for a dying patient and such a phrase should be struck from the parlance of health care workers in this regard. Really it is only another way of saying: 'This patient cannot be cured, I can do nothing.' A better approach is: 'What can I do?'

The doctor, then, working with the dying patient must first reorientate himself. Cure can no longer be held as his only measure of success. Automatic 'patterns' of behaviour in dealing with patients cease to be appropriate. He must develop alternative techniques.

Investigations will need to be limited, certain treatments may need to be stopped because they are no longer controlling the disease and are therefore inappropriate. This will necessitate lengthy explanations to patient and family if they are to be at ease with these changes in management; time must be set aside for giving such explanations and for answering the patient's questions, and those of the family. All too often curative treatment is stopped without explanation; the patient may be well aware of the prognostic significance of this and his dejection is compounded by the thought: 'The doctors have given up on me.'

Even worse, treatment may be continued late into a patient's illness, long after it is inappropriate, because those caring for the patient cannot themselves face the difficulty of a direct explanation to him as to why it is no longer useful. It is easier just to carry on regardless whilst the patient's deteriorating health is denied by all. Time and flexibility are the keys to managing such patients well. The doctor must learn to be flexible in telling patients and families what *they* wish to know rather than what he feels they should be told.

Even if the patient appears to have little to say today, time must be spent in allowing him to make this clear. Above all, the patient must feel free to talk openly and patients will only feel this freedom if the doctor is attentive, concerned and unhurried in his manner (however much else there is to do!).

The doctor must be prepared to befriend his patient, allow him to voice his fears, discuss his anxieties, and spend much time explaining illness and treatment. It may be that he will be humbled more than once by facing the tragedy of his patient's circumstances, or moved to tears of sadness or joy by his patient's comments; such is life, such companionship is itself caring, and will be immediately seen as such by the patient. This relationship between the doctor and dying patient has been compared to that between mother and child, in that, if the doctor openly offers time, concern and explanations, the patient feels a sense of security, protection and trust, which are primordial needs for all of us. The fulfilling of these needs for the patient at the time of death can markedly reduce the pain and suffering of dying. It is the recognition of such needs felt by patients and manifest in many forms, symptoms and problems that is the goal in the hospice approach to the dying person.

Diagnosis

In Britain today malignant disease is the second commonest cause of death in adults, the commonest being cardiovascular disease. In practical terms the dying are those suffering from an inexorably progressive incurable illness, which is ultimately fatal. Cardiovascular illnesses, even in the elderly, are not inexorably progressive and it would be wrong for them to be viewed as such today. Similarly multiple sclerosis sufferers and other handicapped patients should not be seen as 'the dying' or written off. Many such handicaps are compatible with a normal life-span, and rehabilitative care throughout is what is needed for such patients, not 'symptom control'. Thus the commonest diagnosis amongst dying patients will be some form of cancer and amongst these the solid tumours of adult life predominate: these are cancers of bronchus, breast (in women), stomach, colon, pancreas, kidney. Modern treatment can modify the symptomatic course of such diseases considerably, but improves the prognosis little if at all.

The ultimate outcome is virtually uniformly premature death, and a stage is reached in the natural history of all these diseases past which attempts at cure are not only unproductive, but diminish the quality of life remaining for the patient. Some other conditions also give rise to this sort of picture though they are found much less often. These are motor neurone disease, end-stage chronic renal failure and fibrosing alveolitis. Lymphomas, leukaemias and reticuloses – the so called 'diffuse tumours' – have a much better response to treatment than their solid counterparts. Some of these tumours, all rare, are rightly now classed as curable in some patients, but dying patients with these diagnoses are encountered. The doctor caring for the dying patient must have a sound knowledge of oncology – that is the study of malignant disease – and understand the natural history of all these illnesses.

He need not have specialist expertise in the specific treatment of tumours, but he must know and understand the range of therapeutic techniques available and in what circumstances they might usefully be applied so that he can confidently advise patients and relatives and call on other specialist services as needed. It is impossible here to consider in detail the particular illnesses from which patients dying from cancer suffer, but it is worth while to consider further some physical aspects common to such patients.

The primary tumour

In most patients this will have been identified and treated directly by surgery, radiotherapy, chemotherapy or a combination of these. In many instances dying patients show little or no evidence of the primary disease, if the initial treatment has been successful. The problem has become one of disseminated disease and indeed some patients already have metastases at the time of diagnosis.

Primary tumours may recur after treatment either locally or more frequently at distant sites – commonly lungs, liver, bones, lymph nodes and brain. Local recurrence is most common in tumours of the breast, head and neck region. The patient dying with multiple metastatic disease is the commoner occurrence. Some patients with metastases, particularly in bone, may have also received treatment, usually with radiotherapy or chemotherapy, to relieve pain or pressure symptoms, but the patient can no longer be 'cured' because tumours at other sites will remain refractory to treatment. In a minority of patients the primary tumour is so small as to elude detection by simple investigations – the diagnosis is then carcinomatosis from an unknown primary site. The most common sites of minute tumours are bronchus, breast, testis, ovaries, thyroid, stomach and kidney.

This might appear at first an unacceptable level of accuracy in a matter of such importance. Nevertheless, if the primary tumour cannot easily be found and the patient is already suffering from incurable metastatic disease, it is undesirable for him to be subjected to prolonged inpatient care and complex, often uncomfortable investigations for no discernible gain. An uncertain diagnosis is the better choice, and the prognosis is clear. Primary tumours of the brain very rarely spread outside the skull.

Metastatic disease

Lymph nodes   Most forms of cancer spread at first to the group of lymph nodes nearest to their site of origin. Here the tumour cells grow and enlarge. This enlargement, which may be massive, gives rise to pressure effects. In superficial groups of nodes swelling will appear, this occasionally causing skin ulceration. The flow of lymph is obstructed causing lymphoedema in the drainage area of the node group commonly presenting as a swollen upper limb with axillary node destruction from carcinoma of breast or its treatment.

Bones   The skeleton is a frequent site of metastases, which are often extremely painful. Any bones may be affected but most often it is the marrow bones (to which tumour cells are brought in large numbers by the generous blood supply) which are involved: skull, ribs, vertebrae, pelvis and upper humerus and femur. Some cancers show a particular tendency to metastasize to bone (breast, prostate, kidney, thyroid and lung). Sometimes bone is invaded directly by the primary tumour, for instance carcinoma of a bronchus invading ribs.

Bone replaced by tumour growth is weak and pathological fracture may result. The marrow is replaced by tumour cells and this contributes to anaemia.

Hypercalcaemia can also occur due to bone destruction and consequent release of calcium into the blood stream (it may also arise in the absence of bone metastases).

Liver   Liver metastases occur in about one third of patients dying of cancer. They are usually multiple tumour cells, being distributed throughout the liver by both portal and systemic circulations. Sometimes with tumours of the stomach, pancreas and gall-bladder the liver is directly invaded.

The liver involved with cancer enlarges sometimes to fill the whole abdomen. It may be painful and tender. Ascites is usually present and sometimes in such large quantities that aspiration (paracentesis abdominis) is needed to relieve the uncomfortable swelling. Within the liver, bile ducts are obstructed by tumour growth and this causes jaundice. Finally the organ fails, and this may be the cause of death.

Lung   Most commonly lung metastases are blood borne, they may be single or multiple and of variable size. Less often metastatic involvement occurs as the result of lymphatic spread from, for example, the breast. Pleural effusions are a common problem and, if large, will cause dyspnoea. Large deposits in the lung may also obstruct bronchi and cause collapse of peripheral parts of the lung. Infection commonly complicates this picture and combination of collapse, infection and fluid effusion is common, the end result again being dyspnoea and ultimately organ failure.

In considering the principal sites of malignant disease in patients it is worth noting that in any individual patient the full extent of metastatic spread is impossible to define. Occult metastases of ovaries, adrenals and other organs are common and clinical assessments of the number and site of metastases are usually underestimated.

Some effects of wide-spread disease

Cachexia   There is frequently progressive weakness and weight loss in malignant disease. The results in wasting and other biochemical abnormalities are together termed 'cachexia'.

This situation is caused by many factors and bears some relation to the weight of tumour present in the body. The tumour itself consumes vital nutrients and also produces waste products which interfere with normal metabolism. The presence of anorexia, vomiting, ascites, fistula, haemorrhage, infection or ulceration often adds insult to injury and there is increased metabolic rate with protein and calorie malnutrition leading to wasting. Such patients are weak, tire easily and are often depressed; even if food intake is adequate, weight gain is unlikely.

Anaemia   Progressive anaemia is a common finding – malnutrition, recurrent blood loss, altered iron metabolism and infection may all be contributory factors. Progressive marrow infiltration may result in leucoerythroblastic anaemia, and in patients with carcinoma of stomach Vitamin B_{12} deficiency may also occur. A mixed picture is usual. Blood transfusions are sometimes used to relieve (temporarily) the anaemia of malignancy; good results can sometimes be achieved but each patient must be assessed individually. It may be inappropriate to offer transfusion as temporary respite for no useful purpose (as judged, preferably, by the patient) since the treatment once offered has marked psychological effects on patient and family – usually being seen as life sustaining – and thereafter will be requested again even if no longer of use. Thus, facing the issue of the patient's deteriorating health may be postponed, but it cannot ultimately be avoided; conversely transfusion may be a valuable adjunct to radiotherapy and surgery in these patients and is widely used as such.

Prognosis

The prognosis of patients who will benefit from the symptom control approach to management is variable and can never be assessed very accurately. In general it can be said to be less than 6 months. The actual length of estimated life remaining is unimportant. It is necessary for each patient to be assessed individually and the question asked: 'Has the time for terminal care of this patient been reached?'

The doctor needs to consider this point carefully as he must introduce the patient to a new symptom-orientated approach. If the doctor himself feels this approach is inappropriate then the patient is unlikely to be put at his ease. In trying to judge what is appropriate for an individual patient at a specific stage in his illness the doctor must consider several factors:

1　The patient's symptoms.
2　Diagnosis and evidence for progressive disease.
3　Failure of response to curative/conventional treatment.
4　The psychological state of both patient and family.

Positive findings in all of these areas would indicate that the patient is likely to benefit from the care-orientated symptom control approach, but the decision to adopt such an approach may be complicated often by the patient's and his family's psychological attitude being one of denial. Some patients may have severe symptoms but with little or no evidence of active disease.

These people need some support outside hospital, but it is probably more appropriate that this comes from their general practitioner rather than a 'terminal care team'. In other instances patients may have evidence of metastatic disease with few or no symptoms, and it may be that such a patient would be confused by apparently (to him) unnecessary alterations in his care. Some such patients live for many months and it is important for the physician-in-charge to be aware of this; he may wish to offer a little advice, but then have no further involvement until a later date when the patient's difficulties increase.

The patient and his family

The assessment of each patient must be, from the outset, comprehensive. The doctor will have questions which he wishes to ask – although the burden on the patient of this enquiry can be lightened by getting as much information as possible from notes, other staff and relatives beforehand. Equally the patient may have questions which he wishes to ask of the doctor. Much time will need to be given to this initial 'interview', particularly in allowing the patient and family to express their fears. Such fears will not be expressed if the patient and his relatives feel that the doctor is 'too busy' or 'hasn't time' for his problems.

The doctor should, with the information gained from this information and following full physical examination, then have a framework on which to base his treatment, and this will assist the other team members' approach also, if the doctor's notes are accurate. This framework should include:

Patient data   Name, age, address, religion, occupation, own general practitioner's name, hospital attendance if relevant.

Family data   Spouse, children – names, ages, occupations, family illness, recent bereavement.

Physical data   Previous medical history. Present diagnosis, estimated prognosis, previous treatment. Symptoms – pain: site, severity, character. Other symptoms. Physical signs, current medications. Special features, e.g. stoma, wound, fistula, ulcers.

Psychological data   Patient's understanding of own illness and attitude to this. Family's understanding and attitude. Past experience and current priorities.

Home data   Dwelling situation, mobility problems, toilet facilities, phone installed, commode and other aids. District nurse calls, other personnel. Finance/free prescriptions/benefits. Help from voluntary bodies, e.g. Stoma Care Association.

Similarly, once the patient has been assessed initially the doctor must review the situation regularly. It is quite common for a patient to present with many symptoms, the control of which relieves him from much of his burden. His health may then improve and he may live for many months. During this period of 'stability' the doctor must again ask questions: 'Is this patient dying?' If not, then: 'Might more conventional treatment now be of benefit?' This is all part of what should ideally be a continuous process of reassessment.

As an example of this, a patient who eventually died in St Joseph's Hospice was first referred – 'for terminal care' – to the home care service some 4 years before. He was seen and assessed at that time and the home care nurses visited him and his wife for a few weeks. He had metastatic prostatic cancer, but most of his difficulties proved to be due to constipation. This was treated and his health improved considerably. His wife too gained confidence from her contact with the nurses, and 4 weeks after his referral the home care service discharged him back to his general practitioner and hospital outpatients because he was felt to have a good prognosis, and no further symptomatic needs. He lived a perfectly normal life, for one of his age, for a period of 4 years when his general practitioner again referred him because of increasing difficulties. He died a month later. This is an extreme example, but it well illustrates the need for continual review of a patient's circumstances. This approach once adopted is not an irreversible one, and the doctor must prognosticate cautiously and listen to those others involved in the patient's care in deciding what is best for the individual at the particular time.

When discussing prognosis with patients and families a flexible approach is again of prime importance. Many people will have no desire to know 'how long' and it would be wrong to have a fixed idea that they must be told. Others will be curious, and the doctor and other members of the caring team must then be prepared to guide and inform – but at the patient's pace (it may take several days or weeks for the patient's curiosity to be expressed), not their own. In general any attempt at exact prognoses for patients is to be discouraged, especially in the last hours or days of life, when the patient and his family are intensely anxious. Exactness in this regard is unattainable, and if definite prognosis is given the best that will happen is that the patient will die beforehand (he is unlikely to die at the appointed hour) and his family will be left feeling cheated.

At worst he will live past the appointed hour, which will serve only to fuel his loved ones' anxieties at the prolongation of his suffering. In practice the most beneficial approach, for both patient (if he is able to discuss the issue) and relatives, when asked 'How long?' is to reply, 'I don't know,' (no doctor should be afraid to admit this in this context) 'but what we're all interested in is the quality of his remaining life and what we can do to improve it.' (i.e. 'However long it is we must help him to make the most of it.') In my experience any confidence lost by inexactness of prognosis is more than compensated for by the increased assurance of the support, care and guidance offered, and it is rare for patients or relatives not to respond positively to this approach.

Foremost then in gaining the confidence of patient and family is time spent with the patient letting him talk and listening to hear his needs. The second most important factor is to achieve some goal; to reinforce the patient's trust in the doctor's attentiveness to his needs and willingness to search for solutions to his problems. Finding this 'goal' is often very simple. The best approach is often to ask the patient directly: 'What troubles you most of all at the moment?' Clearly, if a patient has severe pain or vomiting or dyspnoea the question will be superfluous, but where all three, and more, symptoms are present at once it is useful to glean the patient's own need and the relevance of each symptom, with the degree of upset it causes him.

It may be that he is stoical about his pain but intensely anxious and alarmed by increasing dyspnoea. His confidence will not, in these circumstances, be increased by pain relief alone. It would be better to tackle the dyspnoea first or both symptoms simultaneously in order to encourage and reassure him. Again, flexibility is vital; the patient may want to tread a different course from that of the doctor and the latter must be prepared to follow his patient's lead (although he can be honest and say if he thinks that the patient's ideas are ill-founded).

When dealing with dying patients the doctor must be aware that the relatives may also to a variable extent become patients. They are certain to have questions, anxieties and fears which if left to fester may assume gigantic proportions. For instance, it is common for the spouse of a patient to be consulting his or her own doctor with various complaints at the time of the loved one's illness (this is also true after bereavement).

Time must also be given to the needs of the relatives; indeed in some instances the close relatives need more time and reassurance than the patient. Equally too, relief of symptoms can be observed very rapidly by the family and, as for the patient, is reassuring and inspires trust.

Good care is based on a trust invested in the doctor and the other members of the caring team. Failure to establish this relationship will leave the doctor unable to help the patient with his fears and may increase his anxieties further, but once established it aids both doctor and patient. Indeed, it is the responsibility of the whole team to develop and foster such a relationship in caring for the patient and his family.

References

Bloom, S W (1965) The Doctor and His Patient: A sociological interpretation, New York Free Press

Hinton, J (1972) Dying, Pelican Books

Hinton, J (1974) Talking with people about to die, British Medical Journal, 1974: 2–25

Lamerton, R (1980) Care of the Dying, Pelican Books

Pritchard, E R (1977) The Family and Death, and Others, Columbia University Press

Saunders, C (ed) (2nd Edn 1981) The Management of Terminal Disease, Edward Arnold

Willis, R A (1973) The Spread of Tumours in the Human Body, Butterworths

Vere, D W (ed) (1978) Topics in Therapeutics: 4, Pitman Medical

CHAPTER 6

MANAGEMENT OF PAIN
JOHN COLLINS, J F HANRATTY
and JOY ROBBINS

WHAT IS PAIN? John Collins

Pain is a protective mechanism for the body; it occurs whenever tissues are damaged and it causes the sufferer to react to remove the painful stimulus. It is, then, a dual sensation; one part being perception the other reaction. In fact this is an over-simplification of an extremely complex phenomenon and it is the purpose of this introduction to explain some of the basic principles upon which our understanding of pain is based.

Acute and chronic pain

It is important to distinguish between acute (or transient) and chronic (persistent) pain. They are perceived differently and give rise to different effects requiring distinct forms of treatment. The former is of secondary importance in, for instance, patients with advanced cancer. It is the latter, chronic pain, which most often affects such people. Usually acute pain is obviously useful, in a protective sense; it is often sharp or pricking in character and may result in rapid physical reaction – as, for example, when the skin is cut with a knife. Frequently the cause is immediately apparent, relief is seen to be near at hand and the pain holds little threat to well-being. Awareness of this in itself aids relief. In contrast chronic pain is a threatening experience rather than a passing event. This sort of pain is usually much less localized – burning, throbbing or aching in character – and since no physical reaction is effective in removing the painful stimulus, the pain tends to get worse rather than better. This causes marked emotional reaction in the sufferer, to whom it represents a great threat to well-being. Indeed it may become such a patient's sole pre-occupation, impossible for him to ignore and pervading every minute of every day. When this point is reached life seems no longer bearable and some patients will request euthanasia as the only perceived form of relief.

Fortunately, as knowledge and expertise improve and disseminate, largely from the hospice movement worldwide, this situation is becoming less common. Sadly, though, even today such patients are found and vigilance is required on the part of all those caring for the terminally ill, in developing skills in the control of pain and in communicating their skills to other workers, to prevent the development of such catastrophic suffering. Particularly the use of 'when required' prescriptions for these patients should be condemned, since this always results in long periods of unrelieved agony, and decreased pain threshold. Some of the differences between acute and chronic pain can be explained on the basis of known physiological mechanisms; others are probably psychological. Clearly both types of pain can coexist in one individual and this must not be forgotten. Not all pains in a patient with, for example, advanced cancer are necessarily due to the cancer itself, and not all the pains caused by cancer will necessarily be identical. These are important points to remember when assessing an individual patient's pain or pains because diagnosis of the cause of the pain is always necessary before appropriate treatment can be planned. For example decubitus and peptic ulcers, and constipation are all potentially painful conditions from which the dying patient may suffer, and all need to be treated specifically rather than with increased prescriptions of strong analgesics.

The pain receptors

The pain receptors in the skin and other tissues are all free nerve endings. They are widespread in the surface layers of the skin and in certain internal tissues such as periosteum, parietal peritoneum and pleura, arterial walls and joint surfaces. Most of the remaining tissues and organs deep within the body are supplied with lesser concentrations of pain nerve endings. Nevertheless, any widespread tissue damage can stimulate large numbers of receptors and cause severe pain from these areas.

The exact mechanism by which these free nerve endings in the tissues are stimulated by 'damage' to the tissue is not known. Research has shown that chemical extracts from damaged tissues can cause pain when introduced into 'normal' tissues and it is almost certain that some chemical substance, which may be Bradykinin, a small protein molecule, released from damaged tissues stimulates the free nerve endings.

This perhaps goes some way toward explaining the action of some non-opiate analgesics. Aspirin, for instance, is known to inhibit some of the effects of Bradykinin and it may diminish its production at the site of injury.

In contrast to most other forms of sensory receptors, pain receptors 'adapt' very little, or not at all, to stimulation. That is, the threshold for excitation of the receptor does not increase with exposure to the stimulus but remains constant, and the pain remains unabated until the stimulus is removed. This contrasts with the adaptation made by the ears to loud sound or the eyes to bright light.

Under certain conditions continued painful stimulus progressively lowers the threshold of excitation, and these receptors become progressively more active with time, i.e. the pain gets worse. This 'negative adaptation' of receptors gives rise to increased sensitivity seen clinically as hyperalgesia or over-sensitivity of an area (usually of skin) wherein pain is elicited by only light touch or pressure.

Pain signals are transmitted from the nerve ending in the tissues to the brain (via the spinal cord) by two different types of nerve fibre. The first and smaller of the two, the delta fibres, conduct impulses very rapidly (3–20 metres per second). The second type C fibres are more sluggish (0.5–2 mps). Therefore a sudden onset of painful stimulus gives a double pain sensation, and a fast sharp or pricking pain is followed a second or so later by a slow burning or aching sensation. The delta fibres quickly apprise the individual of the presence of a damaging stimulus and play an important role in acute pain in initiating immediate reaction to prevent further damage. On the other hand the slow burning sensation delivered by the C fibres tends to become increasingly painful with time. It is this sensation which gives rise to the intolerable suffering of chronic pain.

Spinal cord

Pain fibres of both sorts enter the spinal cord and are there connected via one or two short neurones to long fibres which immediately cross to the opposite side and pass upward to the brain. The intensity of pain signals can be modified as they pass through the interconnections in the spinal cord by simultaneous signals transmitted to the cord from non-pain receptors elsewhere in the body or by signals reaching the spinal cord from the brain. The process is called 'gate control' (theory proposed by Melzack and Wall in 1965) and is the probable explanation for the common experience that pain threshold can be raised or lowered by other stimuli either physical or psychological. It may also, at least partially, explain the mode of action of 'physical analgesics' such as applied heat, acupuncture and transcutaneous electrical nerve stimulation. The theory is that these stimuli activate *non-pain* fibres which are present at interconnections in the spinal cord and block the transmission of signals from *pain* fibres.

The brain and perception of pain

Once received by the brain, pain signals from delta and C type fibres are handled differently. Most of the delta input travels via the thalamus to the cerebral cortex and thus potentially reaches consciousness very quickly.

The C fibre input on the other hand apparently terminates in the thalamus and parts of the brain which together make up what is called the reticular activating system. This system, which is well endowed with opiate receptors, transmits activating signals into all parts of the brain including the hypothalamus, an area known to secrete beta-endorphin – a natural opiate – in response to painful stimuli. Thus, the C fibres, because they excite the reticular activating system, have a very potent effect on the entire nervous system; their sustained activity creates a state of insomnia, anxiety, apprehension and urgency.

Many of the actions of opiate analgesics are attributable to binding of the drugs at specific receptors in the reticular activating systems and other parts of the nervous system. This binding then results in modification of both the sensation and the patient's reaction to it, generating the over-all analgesic effect. The delta fibres might be expected to avoid these modifications since they have few connections in the reticular activating system.

This may explain why opiates give relatively poor relief in certain sorts of pain, for example bone pain and skin trauma where, presumably, delta fibre stimulation predominates.

Recently, naturally occurring compounds called collectively the enkaphalins and endorphins have been discovered. These are produced in the body from various sites in nervous tissue and presumably act as natural analgesics. Acupuncture and transcutaneous electrical nerve stimulation, mentioned earlier in relation to 'gate control', may also act in this way causing increased secretion of endogenous opiates and therefore analgesia. It has been known for some time that some forms of acupuncture analgesic can be reversed by naloxone (Narcan), a specific opiate antagonist, and therefore by inference acupuncture would seem to be at least partly dependent upon endogenous opiate activity for its effect.

Referred pain

Often pain is felt in a part of the body remote from the location of the tissue damage causing it. This is called 'referred pain' and usually it represents pain arising from an internal organ or viscus being referred to an area of the body surface, although it may be referred to another area deep within the body. A knowledge of the types of referred pain is useful in diagnosis of the cause.

Pain is referred because the internal organs themselves cannot be localized and therefore the brain has no direct awareness of the viscera.

The reaction to pain

Even though the threshold for recognition of pain (by receptors) remains roughly constant from person to person, the degree to which each individual reacts to pain varies considerably both between individuals and within one individual in different circumstances. Conditioning, personality and 'gate control' probably all have parts to play in this variability, but more important are factors which can be influenced by those caring for the patient in pain.

Factors which raise pain threshold
reassurance + supportive environment
sleep
rest
distraction
analgesics – particularly opiates
anxiolytics

Factors which reduce pain threshold
fear/isolation
anxiety/depression
anger
insomnia/fatigue

It can thus be seen that there is much to be done for those in pain besides prescribing and administering analgesics.

CONTROL OF PAIN IN TERMINAL CANCER
J F Hanratty

In caring for dying patients where pain is a prominent symptom, the majority will be in the terminal stage of cancer. To achieve successful pain relief, health care workers in this field must have a special understanding of pain and its effect on the sufferer. This section will therefore concentrate specifically on the management of pain due to malignant disease, but much will be applicable to patients dying from other causes who are in pain.

The pain of terminal cancer has no protective or useful purpose. It is not like the acute ephemeral pain such as occurs, for example, if a finger is trapped. It is all-embracing, unremitting and destructive. It clouds the mind and prevents mental concentration and it interferes with social interests and activities. There is also a spiritual component which may prompt such questions as: 'Why me?' – 'What have I done to deserve this?'

The patient's pain threshold may be raised by sympathy, understanding, rest, diversion and a pleasing environment, but most patients will require some analgesic therapy.

Pain analysis

Before dealing with a patient's pain, certain facts must be established. These are: location; severity; onset; course; character; in relation to: movement; meals; bowels; urinary tract; emotions.

Mild pain

Mild pain only needs mild analgesics. Aspirin is a safe and effective minor analgesic for most patients, and it is included in the formulation of a large number of analgesic preparations – mostly in combination with paracetamol and/or codeine. The main disadvantage of aspirin is its tendency to cause gastric irritation in some patients. To overcome this, many formulations have been devised, e.g. enteric-coated, delay release or combinations with antacids. Paracetamol does not have the disadvantage of gastric irritation but may cause constipation. Codeine is a centrally acting narcotic with approximately one tenth the analgesic potency of morphine to which it is metabolized in the body. Dextropropoxyphene is a weak synthetic narcotic similar to methadone.

Some suitable mild analgesics: soluble aspirin 300 mg – 2 every 4 hours; aspirin and codeine (Codis) – 2 every 4 hours; dextropropoxyphene and paracetamol (Distalgesic) – 2 every 4 hours; paracetamol 500 mg every 4 hours; benorylate (Benoral) suspension – 10 ml twice a day; mefenamic acid (Ponstan) 250 mg – 2 three times a day (may cause diarrhoea); dihydrocodeine (DF 118) 30 mg – 2 three times a day (may cause constipation).

Severe pain

As soon as it is apparent that these or similar drugs are ineffective there should be no hesitation in using the stronger opiates.

The use of opiate drugs

1 Give them earlier rather than later in the illness.
2 Give them in sufficient strength.
3 Give them regularly every 4 hours day and night, i.e. not waiting for the pain to recur before giving the next dose.
4 Side effects, e.g. nausea and constipation, should be anticipated.
5 Administer the opiate in a form to ensure absorption.
6 Monitor the dose frequently.
7 The dosage may need to be reduced in the terminal stages, but administration should not be discontinued altogether.

Opiates are frequently withheld for fear of addiction, drowsiness or respiratory depression. Addiction is an irrelevance in terminal illness. Drowsiness, if it does occur, soon wears off. Respiratory depression is rarely any problem and is insignificant in comparison with the overriding benefit the patient obtains from having effective pain control.

The traditional 'Brompton Cocktail' is not a suitable medium for administering opiates as there are so many variants of its formulation, e.g. morphine, diamorphine, cocaine, various phenothiazines and alcoholic flavourings. There is no flexibility in its use, and should an increase in the dose of opiate be needed there is the consequent increase in all the other ingredients with the risk of undesirable side-effects.

Although diamorphine (heroin) is more soluble than morphine, it is relatively unstable in solution. Morphine is usually preferred for oral medication. The approximate oral equivalence of the two drugs is: diamorphine 1.5 times more potent than morphine, e.g. 5 mg diamorphine = 7.5 mg morphine. Cocaine is no longer used as it has no significant beneficial effect.

Morphine sulphate given orally in an appropriate dose (depending on what medication the patient has been having previously) is the most effective introduction of an opiate. A customary start for a patient previously inadequately relieved by non-narcotic drugs would be 5 mg or 10 mg every 4 hours: morphine sulphate 5 mg with syrup or appropriate flavouring as required; chloroform water to 10 ml – dose – 10 ml every 4 hours. The strength of each dose of the morphine may be increased by 5 mg a day until the dose reaches 20 mg and thereafter 10 mg each day until effective pain control is achieved. Most patients obtain pain relief with doses in the region of 30 mg morphine sulphate 4-hourly although doses in excess of 150 mg 4-hourly are occasionally needed.

It is essential to ensure that the patient takes the medication every 4 hours throughout the 24 hours, although a larger dose at bedtime or the addition of a slow release morphine tablet (e.g. MST Continus) at 10 p.m. sometimes obviates the administration of a dose during the night.

Should the patient be unable to take oral medication (e.g. because of vomiting or dysphagia or weakness) the opiate may then be administered per rectum in the form of morphine suppositories. These are available in strength of 15 mg, 30 mg and 60 mg, and provided there is no rectal or bowel pathology preventing administration, nor pelvic pathology hindering absorption, this method of administration is almost as effective as by mouth. As with oral medication, the drug must be given every 4 hours. Oxycodone (Proladone) suppositories are also available and are equivalent to 20 mg of morphine. The duration of Proladone as suppository is longer and should therefore be given about every 6 or 8 hours.

If oral and rectal administration are impossible, the opiate will have to be given by injection. Diamorphine is clearly the drug of choice for injections as its greater solubility enables larger doses to be given in a smaller volume of fluid – e.g. 1 g morphine needs 20 ml of water for solution, whereas 1 g diamorphine needs 2 ml of water for solution. By injection diamorphine is twice as potent as morphine – e.g. 5 mg diamorphine = 10 mg morphine. Morphine and diamorphine are twice as potent by injection, therefore when transferring from oral to injection therapy the dose should be halved.

Patients unsuitable for treatment by oral or rectal medication usually require 4-hourly injections, which may be unsettling or even distressing. The need for regular injections can be obviated by the use of the Greaseby Dynamics Portable Syringe Driver (MS16). A 24-hour dose of the medication – usually diamorphine and prochlorperazine (Stemetil) – is drawn into a 10 ml syringe to which a cannula with a butterfly needle is attached. The syringe is fitted into the driver which is set to compress the syringe at a steady rate and empty the syringe in 24 hours. The butterfly needle is inserted subcutaneously in the supraclavicular region and the driver fits snugly into a sling under the arm. Excellent and continuous pain control is achieved with this method often with a smaller total dose of medication. The syringe is re-charged each day, and the needle site is altered after 48 hours. *Further information is given in the Note on page 75.*

Other opiate drugs with morphine equivalence are: dipipanone hydrochloride 10 mg and cyclizine 30 mg (Diconal) = 5 mg morphine; papaveretum 10 mg (Omnopon) = 5 mg morphine; phenazocine 5 mg (Narphen) = 25 mg morphine; levorphanol 1.5 mg (Dromoran) = 8 mg morphine; dextromoramide 5 mg (Palfium) = 15 mg morphine; methadone 5 mg (Physeptone) = 7.5 mg morphine; slow release morphine (MST Continus) given twice a day – available 3 strengths = 10/30/60 mg morphine; buprenorphine hydrochloride (Temgesic sublingual) 0.2 mg = 5 mg morphine. As this drug is a partial morphine antagonist, it should not be given in conjunction with other opiates.

Palfium is too short-acting (1–2 hours) for routine use, but it may be used as a supplement, e.g. before some potentially painful procedure. Physeptone has a long half life and a tendency to cumulation – it is not advisable for regular continuous use, but may be helpful as a nocturnal supplement.

Pethidine and pentazocine (Fortral) are not suitable drugs for the severe pain of terminal cancer as their action is too short-lasting and they have a tendency to cause confusional side-effects.

Side-effects of opiate drugs Nausea and vomiting are controlled by administering prochlorperazine (Stemetil) 5 mg every 4 hours or haloperidol (Serenace) 0.5 mg twice a day. Domperidone (Motilium) 10 mg three times a day is also useful. The nausea and vomiting are often initiation reactions and wear off after a few days enabling the anti-emetics to be reduced or even withdrawn.

Constipation needs to be anticipated. Danthron (Dorbanex Forte syrup) 10 ml daily is useful for this. Other side effects, such as sweating, dizziness, confusion, are not common and usually subside after a few days.

Opiates are the most useful drugs for combating pain but other therapies may be indicated to control special types of pain; there may also be different types of pain due to a variety of causes acting at the same time. It is helpful therefore to analyse the pain.

Specific types of pain

Visceral pain (e.g. colic) may respond to dicyclomine (Merbentyl) or propantheline (Pro-Banthine). Continued use of these drugs may lead to troublesome side-effects such as dry mouth, and urinary retention.

Bone pain This usually arises from bony metastases arising particularly from primary cancer of lung, breast or prostate – although other tumours may also metastasize in bone. Non-steroid anti-inflammatory drugs act as antiprostaglandins within the bone and are often very effective in reducing bone pain: benorylate (Benoral) 10 ml twice a day; indomethacin (Indocid) 25 mg or 50 mg three times a day, also as sustained release tablet (Indocid-R) 75 mg at night, and as suppositories 100 mg twice a day; flurbiprofen (Froben) 50–100 mg three times a day. All of these may occasionally cause gastric irritation.

Steroids in the form of enteric-coated prednisolone 10 mg twice a day are also very useful for bone pain. Palliative radiotherapy should be considered if the patient has not already received the maximum dose. Immobilization is occasionally helpful although patients do not usually welcome a plaster or splints.

Muscle spasm – may respond to: baclofen (Lioresal) 5 mg three times a day increasing to 20 mg three times a day; dantrolene (Dantrium) 25 mg three times a day increasing to 100 mg three times a day; diazepam (Valium) 5 mg three times a day. Nocturnal cramps are occasionally helped by quinine sulphate 300 mg at night. Clonazepam (Rivotril) 0.5

mg three times a day increasing slowly to 2 mg three times a day, is effective for myoclonus especially in uraemia. Physiotherapy is often very helpful.

Nerve compression   The severe neuritic pains from nerve compression can only be effectively relieved by reducing the compression or ablating the nerve. Sometimes significant relief is obtained by using diuretics and steroids to reduce tissue fluid and inflammation.

Transcutaneous nerve stimulation using a portable high frequency, low voltage stimulator, e.g. 'Tiger Pulse', is sometimes dramatically effective – especially for brachial plexus lesions. The optimum siting of the electrodes and adjustment of the stimulator may not be obtained at once and there is scope for trial, with the help of the patient to obtain the best result.

Nerve blocks – peripheral, sympathetic, epidural or intrathecal – may be needed occasionally, and the help of an expert, usually at a Pain Clinic, may be required. The patient must be warned beforehand that the treatment may result in permanent partial or even complete paresis of a limb, or sometimes urinary or bowel incontinence. Some patients feel that permanent loss of mobility or control is too high a price to pay for complete pain relief.

Intractable pain may need neurosurgery, e.g. cordotomy or thalamotomy; pituitary ablation may also be considered. These extreme therapies are rarely necessary.

Raised intracranial pressure   causing severe headaches or neck-rigidity can often be relieved by dexamethasone 4 mg four times a day. After several weeks the dose is reduced, otherwise Cushingoid features will develop. The intracranial pressure will eventually rise again as the tumour grows but the few weeks or months of relief are well worth achieving.

Diuretics are not usually of any benefit for raised intracranial pressure.

Lymphoedema   The pain of distension and the weight of a massively swollen limb can often be diminished by intermittent compression using Jobst pressurized cushion. Dexamethasone 8 mg daily is often effective.

Infection and ulceration   Pain from these causes should be treated by using appropriate antibiotics and by drainage of any abscess which has formed. Povidone-iodine (Betadine) preparations are useful for sores, ulcers and fungating lesions.

Other causes of pain   A dying patient may suffer great distress from conditions quite unrelated to the terminal disease. Toothache, dyspepsia, musculoskeletal conditions, thrombophlebitis, constipation, haemorrhoids, various infections are just some of the potentially painful conditions which may occur. They should respond to specific treatment and such treatment should not be withheld just because the patient is dying.

Note—Syringe driver

The Syringe Driver Type MS16, made by Greaseby Dynamics Ltd, is compact, lightweight, and is designed to drive home the barrel of a syringe at a predetermined rate with the aid of an electronic timer. The instrument is easily held in a shoulder holster, and a 60 cm cannula runs from the syringe, ending in a butterfly needle which is inserted subcutaneously in convenient site, e.g. the suprascapular region.

In a clinical trial (1981) the Syringe Driver was used at St Joseph's Hospice on a total of 65 patients for the continuous subcutaneous infusion of diamorphine mixed with prochlorperazine (Stemetil) or other anti-emetics as a means of controlling severe pain in patients suffering from advanced cancer.

The appropriate daily dose of diamorphine and prochlorperazine (Stemetil) was determined and drawn into a 10 ml syringe which was fitted into the Driver and this was set to compress the barrel at a rate of 2 mm per hour, which meant that the syringe would be empty in 25 hours.

When starting to use the Driver a loading dose of 1 ml, i.e. one tenth of the daily dose, is given intramuscularly before the Driver is activated.

Experience in the use of the Syringe Driver (65 patients)*

1   Indurations may develop at the needle site. These are due to reaction to the phenothiazines which are added as anti-emetics. 20% of patients receiving prochlorperazine (Stemetil) via the Driver developed indurations. Methotrimeprazine (Veractil) and chlorpromazine

---

*Annual Report, St Joseph's Hospice, Hackney, for year April 1980–April 1981

(Largactil) were considered to be responsible for indurations in a few patients. No local reactions have resulted from metoclopramide (Maxolon) or cyclizine. Diamorphine alone has never caused any local reaction. Hyaluronidase (Hyalase) was not effective in preventing these phenothiazine indurations. If indurations do develop the phenothiazine being used should be stopped.

2   The needle site is usually changed every 48 hours.

3   Diamorphine 24-hour dose has ranged from 60 mg to 480 mg.

4   Average length of time in use was 12 days; maximum 16 weeks.

5   Pain control was achieved in 100% of cases once the optimum dose was found – this was usually immediate but occasionally adjustments were necessary over 2–3 days.

6   Nausea and vomiting were relieved completely in 70% of cases. The remaining 30%, while still vomiting, had considerably less distress from nausea.

7   20% of patients were so effectively relieved from pain and vomiting that it was possible to resume oral medication.

Following the success of this trial, the Syringe Driver has been used regularly in the Hospice and several hundred patients have had excellent pain control by this means.

Summary

	Male	Female
Number of patients treated—	186	258
No pain, or minor pain relieved by mild analgesics—	74(39.8%)	100(38.8%)
Needed opiates at some time—	112(60.2%)	158(61.2%)
Needed morphine 30 mg or more 4-hourly at some time—	65(35%)	73(28.3%)
Treated with diamorphine via the Syringe Driver—	17(9.1%)	10(3.9%)

The need for prescribing opiates even in small doses was regarded as indicative of significant pain. The need for 30 mg or more of morphine 4-hourly was indicative of severe pain.

References

Hanratty, J F (1981) Control of Distressing Symptoms in the Dying Patient, St Joseph's Hospice

Saunders, C M (ed) (1978) The Management of Terminal Disease, Edward Arnold

Twycross, R G (1974) Clinical experience with diamorphine in malignant disease, International Journal of Clinical Pharmacology Therapy and Toxicology: 184

Twycross, R G (1977) Care of the terminal patient, in B A Stoll (Editor) Breast Cancer Management, William Heinemann Medical Books

NURSING MANAGEMENT OF THE PATIENT WITH PAIN
Joy Robbins

The nurse has a powerful and responsible position with regard to pain. She is often the key person to resolve whether the patient's pain gets better or worse, since nurses provide a continuous service to patients and are thus in a position to convey an accurate picture to the doctor of the pattern of the pain. This entails developing skills of observation in which all aspects of the symptoms are perceived and understood.

Attitudes and communications

If the nurse is to help the patient she must accept that pain is a subjective experience. Any sense by the patient that the reality and degree of his pain is doubted will have a detrimental effect. Depression will occur, if not already present, and this is likely to intensify the pain, since tension and depression are interrelated. A guiding principle should be *'Pain is whatever the experiencing person says it is'* (McCaffery 1983). This is fundamental to nursing the patient effectively and is linked with the conviction that pain is affected by the emotions which may be experienced by the dying patient, notably fear. Indeed, fear of pain that will become increasingly intolerable is not uncommonly the most prominent feature in many people's expectation of dying. When the dying patient is actually suffering from unrelieved and severe pain, this becomes a vicious circle with fear exacerbating the pain.

In assessing the needs of a dying patient, the ability to recognize cues regarding pain experience is crucial. There must be time to listen to the patient's description of his pain, to watch for non-verbal signs, for example facial expression, posture, and sounds such as moaning, rapid breathing or sighing.

Sometimes the nurse will experience inward distress at witnessing pain not yet adequately relieved in a dying person. In such a difficult situation where, despite efforts by the caring team, the problem is not yet resolved, there may even be a temptation for the carer to avoid the patient because of these painful emotions.

The nurse needs to develop a positive attitude towards the availability of resources to control pain. These include not only the use of drugs and various therapies which the doctor will initiate and the nurse will be responsible for maintaining, but also a number of other means of relieving pain which the nurse can operate alone.

Some methods of pain relief

It must be accepted that the nature of pain, its causes and relief are not fully understood; therefore it is necessary to work *with* the patient to alleviate his pain. New information is constantly unfolding in this field and can enhance understanding of how to manage individual pain control. For instance, it is now recognized that the use of placebos will relieve actual physical pain, and that this does not mean that the patient is a malingerer.

Being with the patient

Simply staying with the patient can contribute to pain relief. This is because anxiety and other distressing emotions may be lessened because of a feeling of confidence in the patient that he is not left alone, especially with anticipatory fears that the pain will return.

It also gives the patient the opportunity to gain relief from some of the mental pain which may be afflicting him, and he may choose to unburden himself to the nurse who is giving her company. Thoughts of impending loss of everything that life holds for him, terror at the idea of death coming in a violent manner, or a sense of frustration at what seems in retrospect a life containing little tangible achievement call for compassionate and unhurried listening. 'Physical and mental suffering are closely interwoven and a division into bodily and mental pain is an artificial one' (Lamerton 1980).

Achieving comfort of position

The patient may find it difficult to achieve a comfortable position in bed or chair, due to emaciation and thus pressure on bony prominences. Or oedema may be present, causing painful tension of swollen limbs or abdomen. The presence of pressure sores will add to the problem. In patients with cancer, the presence of bony secondary deposits calls for very careful handling by the nurse both to avoid causing pain and also because of the risk of pathological fractures.

The patient himself and the relatives may have found the best way of sitting or lying to avoid pain, and the most comfortable arrangement of pillows, and the nurse should accept their advice. A variety of positions may be adopted, and plenty of pillows should be available; the large triangular pillow is often valued. Patients with neck lesions need special attention; sometimes a cervical collar is helpful, or small neck pillows. Other aids to comfort in bed, or sitting in a chair, which are commonly used in nursing for many types of patient can all be of value to the dying patient in helping to relieve pain.

The patient with spinal metastases or spinal cord lesion will need particular attention. A firm-based bed is essential, as is careful positioning of limbs to prevent contractures. Some form of paralysis may be present and therefore all these points regarding position are of great importance. If the paralysis is of recent occurrence the patient will probably be anxious and frustrated by loss of function, and need a sympathetic and positive approach from his carers. The help of a physiotherapist will be an asset to advise on suitable exercises and aids to support of the paralysed limb. These include ripple beds, sheepskins to sit on or place under heels, and footstools.

Dealing with painful skin and mucous membranes

Since all systems of the body are linked together, the dying patient will have a number of physical discomforts to contend with, some of which may cause severe pain, and not be directly caused by his main disease. The skin is a potent guide to the state of an individual's health, and inevitably is at risk in the deteriorating dying body. Pressure sores may arise, despite care, or gravitational ulcers in the patient with cardiovascular disease. Preventive measures having failed, nursing care must be planned to minimize the pain and further break-down of the skin and underlying tissue. This will require judicious topical medication, and relief of pressure on the area.

A painful mouth is very common, and should always be anticipated in the dying patient by frequent topical care, using any special medication prescribed by the doctor. Severe ulceration with haemorrhage may occur, particularly in patients with leukaemia or end-stage renal failure, and is very painful. Dryness of the mouth adds to the discomfort, and the nurse should use all measures to relieve this, realizing that the patient may not be able to draw attention to the problem.

The presence of haemorrhoids is another condition which can cause much pain and misery to the dying patient, exacerbated if the patient tries to pass hard stools. Here, prevention of constipation is a serious responsibility on the nurse's part, to avoid this largely unnecessary pain. If haemorrhoids, or anal fissure, are present, local application of suitable ointment or analgesic rectal suppositories should be used.

In women, the vulva may be a site for tenderness and pain if, for instance, a malignant lesion is present. Or a rectovaginal fistula will also result in an inflamed mucosa and be very painful because of the excretions passing over it. The pain is further compounded in the conscious patient by embarrassment and anxiety because of the site involved, and the unpleasant smell which is often present. Here, the tact and gentleness of the nurse is all-important. Local treatment to soothe the inflammation and to maintain hygiene is required, and care that the level of analgesic drugs that the patient is receiving is at an appropriate level to aim at controlling the pain.

The bladder mucosa may become inflamed; cystitis is quite a common and very painful condition. Antibiotic therapy is usually prescribed unless the patient is near death, and the nurse should also take the usual steps of seeing that the patient is taking as much fluid as possible, and handle an indwelling catheter with scrupulous care to avoid further infection.

The patient may have an open wound which is extensive and painful. Malignant skin lesions, such as fungating carcinoma of breast, are unpleasant both for the patient and the nurse. Secondary infection is likely, and offensive odour. This is another example of pain with both a physical and mental component, needing analgesic drugs to control the pain, plus local dressings, and some means of suppressing the odour such as an aerosol spray used in the room.

Headache

A dying patient may suffer from an occasional headache like anyone else, which clears up quickly following administration of a mild analgesic such as aspirin.

Headaches may, however, have a grave cause such as a brain tumour, or occur in end-stage renal failure. Here the headaches will be intense, prolonged and occur at frequent intervals. The pressure building up within the skull is due to excess cerebrospinal fluid and, in the case of a tumour, actual increase in size of the space-occupying lesion.

Temporary relief can often be obtained by giving large doses of steroid drugs which will reduce oedema in and around the tumour, and thus the intracranial pressure. Unfortunately, a decision eventually has to be made as to how long this palliative treatment should continue.

Whether the headache is from a benign or malignant cause, the nurse can help to relieve the pain by using such time-honoured simple remedies as cold compresses to the forehead, shading the patient's eyes from bright lights and providing a quiet atmosphere.

Use of relaxation and distraction techniques

Relaxation can be defined as a state of freedom from both anxiety and skeletal muscle tension. The dying patient with pain is likely to be anxious and tense, which lowers his pain threshold. Simple techniques, such as getting the patient into as comfortable a position as possible and instructing him to close his eyes and breathe rhythmically and deeply, can be used by the nurse. Sometimes soft slow music may help, and act as a distraction from the pain.

Distraction as a non-invasive pain relief method is a kind of sensory shielding, a protecting of oneself from the pain sensation by focusing on and increasing the clarity of sensations unrelated to pain (McCaffery 1983). The nurse who wishes to try this method needs to know her patient well enough to judge what distraction would be most likely to help. For instance, if the patient is very keen on sporting events, the topic could be introduced and discussed for a brief period. Music has already been mentioned, and the use of visual images such as showing the patient a series of pictures likely to interest him is another example.

This whole field of non-invasive pain relief methods is a complex one, and is arousing a good deal of interest for patients with chronic pain, including those in a terminal stage of illness. Cutaneous stimulation is another method which includes some ancient techniques, such as use of heat and cold applications to the body, massage and counterirritants, and transcutaneous electric nerve stimulation. A further step, where the skin is actually penetrated, is acupuncture.

Some of these ideas may be used with benefit to the dying patient by the nurse and doctor working together or singly according to the degree of sophistication favoured. Special training is needed before using certain relaxation and distraction techniques, and details of these are beyond the scope of this book.

Administration of drugs for control of pain

Since this is the main way of controlling physical pain, it is considered fitting to end this section by emphasizing again the crucial role of the nurse in the matter. The basic principles of safe administration of drugs are, of course, as important here as in any situation, especially as most of the drugs used will be opiates, i.e. Controlled Drugs.

There are other aspects which need special mention:

1   Oral medication is used as much as possible, and the dying patient often needs help with this towards the end, when weakness is increasing and muscle co-ordination is difficult. An unhurried approach is essential.

2   Close monitoring of the effects of the drug will mainly fall on the nurse. If the pain is unrelieved or has re-appeared before the next dose is due, this must be reported as soon as possible to the doctor so that action can be taken to improve control of the pain. It is important that the nurse checks the effect of the drug about half an hour after it has been administered, and then at least half an hour before the next dose is due.

3   When death is near, it should be remembered that if opiates have been given regularly to control pain, they must continue to be given even if the patient becomes semicomatose. If this principle is not followed and an opiate is suddenly discontinued, there may be withdrawal reactions, and the patient may experience pain even though unable to communicate verbally. Drugs which hitherto have been taken orally will now have to be administered by suppositories or injection. The dose of the drug will continue to need careful assessment by the nurse and the doctor. Sometimes the amount may be reduced but occasionally there may be evidence of increasing pain requiring larger doses of opiates.

Patients and their relatives need to be assured that putting up with the pain is contrary to the goal being aimed for, and that there is no question of the patient being considered cowardly or ungrateful if he gives an accurate picture of inadequate relief. The qualified nurse also has a responsibility to educate her junior colleagues, e.g. student nurses, in the proper approach to pain control. Paying lip service to the principles is insufficient; attitudes are more often 'caught, not taught'.

The nurse who acts compassionately and intelligently with her medical colleagues in striving to reach the ideal situation of complete pain control renders a considerable service to her dying patients.

References

Hayward, J (1981) Information – A prescription against pain, Royal College of Nursing – Research Project

Hinton, J (1972) Dying, Pelican Books

Hockey, L (1981) Recent Advances in Nursing – 1: Current Issues in Nursing, Churchill Livingstone

Lamerton, R (1980) Care of the Dying, Pelican Books

McCaffery, M (1983) Nursing the Patient in Pain, Harper & Row

Raiman, J (1981) Responding to pain, Nursing, November

CHAPTER 7

COMMUNICATIONS WITH PATIENT AND FAMILY
BERYL MUNNS

Introduction

'Communication is so important with people like us; if you can get through to someone it automatically lifts the fear.' This view was expressed by Mrs Jones shortly before she died. She had been ill for a long time, was aware of her prognosis and had experienced pain and fear. Her understanding of the concept of communication was comprehensive, in that she saw it as part of all human interaction, and as including not only words, but tone, gesture, touch, sound and the use of many symbols. Mrs Jones realized too that if communication was to be meaningful then those at both ends of the communication channel needed to be able to understand each other and to be competent and willing in their interaction.

Since there are so many elements involved it is not surprising that effective communication is difficult to achieve. Misunderstanding is a common experience in everyday life. This situation cannot be afforded in nursing, when the welfare of patients is at stake, and no field is more important in this respect than that of the care of dying patients. Here good care depends to a great extent on really efficient communication between nurse, patient, and the family, and within the whole health care team. Yet it is just in this area of care that communication difficulties or barriers arise to make achievement that much harder.

This chapter discusses these extra barriers, whilst recommending a general study of human interaction, on which subject several books have been written. It then examines some of the messages that are communicated to patients and their families and the means by which they are conveyed.

Barriers on the nurse's side

Several barriers can arise on the nurse's side. They stem from attitudes and values that are not entirely negative in themselves but suited more to one situation than another, and which may hinder communication in the care of the dying. The nurse acquires these attitudes during her socialization as a member of society and during her professional training and experience.

Society's barriers

In the twentieth century members of Western societies are not well prepared to consider death and dying, except in an impersonal way as presented by the media. In previous eras the frequency of death in early life meant that dying was not divorced from everyday family awareness, and religious teaching often centred round this theme. Therefore people learned to accept the end of life as well as the beginning.

Today people are healthier and live longer; greater population mobility splits the extended family so that there is less contact with the older family members. It is therefore possible to reach adulthood having had little association with death or bereavement. The result is that the very natural fear of death becomes enlarged and unacceptable. People become embarrassed in the presence of the terminally ill patient and his family. A barrier of defence is set up and the coping method chosen is one of avoidance whenever decently possible.

The barrier of the value given to cure

Over the past years there have been many wonderful advances in medicine and so it is often possible to think in terms of cure. Other discoveries mean that the ultimate – prevention – may now be achieved. Consequently there is great emphasis on prevention and cure. Indeed research has found that many persons enter the health care professions motivated by the goal of cure. When this is no longer possible then there is frequently a deep sense of failure.

It is unrealistic, however, to think in terms of cure for large sections of patients who are chronically sick, or in the terminal stages of disease. The problem is that with the sense of failure there is often the feeling that no clear or worthwhile goal is left. This seems somewhat strange in nursing, which is a caring rather than curing profession, but this attitude contributes to the embarrassment some nurses feel with dying patients, which they meet by cutting down the time spent in patient contact.

The answer to this situation is the recognition that new and more appropriate goals may be adopted, which can bring great comfort to patients and their families, and these will be discussed later in this chapter. When these goals are met the aimless feeling need no longer cloud the view of those working with patients for whom cure is no longer possible.

The barrier of stereotype

The system of viewing patients within diagnostic categories has developed over the years. It is useful in that specialization brings greater skills to care and this labelling provides a form of shorthand for indicating the types of observations, precautions and treatment needed. It provides little understanding, however, of persons as individuals. The effect may be negative in that when another form of label is applied – that of 'dying' – all the inhibitions surrounding the subject become attached to the patient.

It is often necessary to recognize, of course, that a terminal stage of illness has been reached, but this knowledge should not diminish the view of the patient as an individual. John, policeman, husband, father of four, supporter of widowed mother, athlete, reader of thrillers need not become John, dying, needs to be kept comfortable. Whilst John remains within himself much the same, or perhaps a little enlarged because his situation has given him the opportunity to explore his feelings or develop an interest that he has not had time for before, professionals can see him as diminished. If communications are based on the narrower view then the goals of care lack imagination. This situation calls for correction of view based on sensitive personal communications with John and his family.

The barrier of activity

There are many reasons for an emphasis on physical activity. Nursing uses a variety of practical skills and the importance given to rules of procedure is necessary to ensure safe practice. Staff shortage over the years has meant that nurses have considered it necessary to give priority to essential practical tasks such as making beds. It is not surprising therefore that nursing has often been task oriented and that nurses tend to feel guilty when 'just' quietly sitting talking to a patient.

Today through the Nursing Process we are beginning to use in a systematic way the knowledge that has been intuitively felt for years, namely that good nursing care can only result from an understanding of the patient as a whole person in a social situation. This knowledge must be obtained through good communication with the patient, his family and with other professional people who now share his support or who have been involved with him in the past.

Sometimes it is necessary to be still, to listen, and to share with the patient; at other times a quality of listening and responsiveness whilst undertaking the practical task will be sufficient. However achieved, meaningful communication is vitally important in the care of dying patients where there is a battle with fear, anxiety and physical symptoms such as pain and nausea. These cannot always be separated from each other. The sharing of fear may of itself reduce tension and relieve pain or point the way to some new beneficial approach. Therefore the value placed on practical activity should not be allowed to bar communication, which could meet the need more efficiently than a multiplicity of tasks.

The barrier of the value of secrecy

This value can create a great barrier between nurse and patient, for nurses are often placed in a very difficult position when they are aware that the patient has not been told of his prognosis. They tend to cope with a bright and rather brusque manner, and with avoidance behaviour, to discourage awkward questions which they feel they should not answer.

However this type of reaction does convey something to patients. Mrs Smith returned from theatre where it had been discovered that she had an inoperable carcinoma. Long before her doctor told her about this, she had correctly assessed the behaviour of the staff and knew of her situation. This meant that at that time of weakness she was presented with a fearsome knowledge without the reassurance, comfort and support that should go with it. Many patients may be in this position; a recent survey of 482 patients admitted to a hospice in a terminal condition found that over 20% knew or were suspicious of their situation despite having been given no clear information on the subject. This is not to suggest that this was all due to the behaviour of professionals, but silence of staff and family played a part.

To be told the truth is, however, a traumatic experience for nearly everyone, calling for inner resources which, according to the patient's condition, may be available more at one time than another. It is therefore right that caution should be exercised as to when to tell and how much to tell and what way to tell it. A policy of many is, not to force unwelcome news upon an unsuspecting and unready patient but to be very sensitive to his cues indicating desire for knowledge, so that his requirements may be met at the right time and in the right depth. An enquiring patient has a right to know. He may then be able to manage his remaining days as he wishes, perhaps seek to achieve some special goal, make arrangements for dependents or explore spiritual issues.

The decision 'to tell' is an important one and needs to be based on sound information provided by the care team. The nurse, particularly a junior one, is often important here, for she has the greatest contact with the patient. Whilst she is caring for him the patient often communicates his fears and poses slanted questions. These can be relayed to senior team members. The patient may ask direct questions and it can be quite natural to reflect the question back – for example, 'You seem to be concerned about . . . . . . would you like to talk about it with someone who has more details, Sister or Doctor?' The request can then be passed on promptly.

The secrecy barrier means that nurse/patient communications are often surrounded by fear on both sides and become unnatural. If the nurse is prepared to meet questions rather than avoid them she will be less likely to convey her awkwardness and fear to the patient. If her sensitivity to the patient's cues for knowledge has enabled her to play a part in his receiving the right information, she may well be rewarded by seeing a release from tension on his part and a greater trust in relationships. She will then no longer be afraid to give herself to patients in meaningful communication.

The barrier of hierarchy

Nurses have always been very conscious of hierarchies, both in the institution and within each nursing team. Channels of command help to provide an orderly setting for care but can be restrictive in that the junior members of staff, who often see most of the patient, have little influence in the decisions that are made on behalf of the patient.

This situation is not helpful in the area of terminal care where a very broad spectrum of factors is involved; those that are physical, psychosocial and spiritual. The team has to be multidisciplinary and include all the members of each discipline. Each nurse needs to value her potential to contribute to team knowledge and decision making, and must be prepared to express her own objective professional opinion as well as to communicate the patient's feelings and wishes.

Good communications within the team, based on mutual respect, will enhance the effectiveness of care, and the resulting atmosphere of unity will be sensed by patients who will then be encouraged to enter into trusting relationships.

Towards breaking nurse barriers

It would be foolish to assume that long-held attitudes and fears may be instantly removed in pursuit of better nurse/patient communications, but the following suggestions may help to initiate the process.

1 *Be gentle and patient with yourself.* Those who have had long experience in the field of terminal care recognize that it takes many months, perhaps up to two years, for staff to feel comfortable and confident working with dying patients. It may become less difficult very gradually, or there may be more of a sudden break-through which relates to some specific experience or achievement with a patient.

2 *Seek to understand your feelings.* Sharing them with other members of the team helps, as does not being afraid to express the emotions that will arise. Are any of the barriers just discussed yours? It is difficult to come to terms with the situation of patients before one has honestly examined one's own feelings about personal mortality.

3 *Seek to learn* as much as possible about the processes of dying. Understanding then brings the knowledge of how best to cope with patients' problems whether they be physical or emotional. Success helps to bring confidence. Many books have been written on the subject and amongst the most inspiring are the accounts of people who are facing dying. Through them we realize something of the feelings involved and, most important, that this experience can have positive as well as negative aspects. This encourages the search for extra goals that centre around quality of life.

4 *Plan goals.* Communication is rather circular in effect. We share

some time with patients and begin to understand them as individuals. This knowledge helps us to look for positive goals, based on their values, and we are then able to communicate on a deeper level. Some goals are more positive than others. For example 'Tender Loving Care' (TLC) has often been used by the health care professions to denote the attention needed by the chronically sick or terminally ill patient. It suggests gentleness and compassion without which there would not be the insight to use skills. It also suggests endeavour to keep the patient as comfortable and free from unpleasant complications as possible. It does not necessarily emphasize the achievement of other and extra goals that may greatly add to the patient's quality of life.

Mrs Peters, a young patient, was struggling to finish knitting a scarf and was finding it difficult to cope with the thick wool and large needles. She could not manage to 'cast off'. A passing nurse spent a few minutes doing this for her while she explained the method. Mrs Peters' face lit up with pleasure and she said, 'I have never in all my life had a finished piece of knitting.' She went on with great enthusiasm to make another scarf and this time completed it herself. This may seem a relatively small achievement but it added an extra quality to her last days.

Sensitive communication with patients helps the nurse, as part of a team, to provide the right environment for individuals to meet their own needs, whether they result from activity or from quiet thought. When, in a caring environment, patients are seen to renew relationships or turn from fear and bitterness to peaceful trust, the reward to the nurse is great. It heightens the awareness of the potential of communication in all its forms and sustains the nurse through the many difficulties she experiences.

Barriers on the patient's side

Patients often experience factors that make effective communication more difficult for them. These may relate to the patient's expectations of his role in the ward situation, to physical and emotional states, as well as to the environment provided for him.

'Taking the sick role'

'Taking the sick role' is a phrase used to describe a set of attitudes and behaviour adopted by people when they become ill, particularly when they are admitted to an institution such as a hospital. It is helpful to patients in that they are expected to opt out of the responsibilities of life and take a passive resting role, leaving large and small decisions to others. It is easy to encourage this legitimate behaviour because it assists the running of wards and is also necessary for safety. Essentially the patient relinquishes his autonomy for his own welfare and that of others.

When patients are in a terminal stage of illness the situation is somewhat different. They are not giving up in the short term for a long-term gain; the present is the only time that they have for making wide-ranging decisions for their own lives and that of others. Their state also demands that every effort be made to bring their own values of quality into their daily lives. In order for this to be achieved patients must feel invited to communicate their thoughts and wishes. If, however, the 'sick role' expectations are carried over from previous experiences, they will be inhibited.

Through their interest and concern for each patient as a unique individual, nurses can help patients feel free to express their feelings, so that their needs may be met, in that they may be supported in their own decision making.

Physical condition

However much the patient may wish to communicate with those around, his ability may be limited by his physical condition. He may have a tumour of the larynx, for example. Many patients in a terminal stage of disease are elderly, as are relatives, and so they may suffer from diminished sight or hearing. Loss of any sense makes it harder in a general way to send or receive messages, since the senses depend upon each other to produce total pictures.

Meaningful communication also requires clear perception and this may be clouded where there is cerebral disturbance or the presence of various combinations of drugs. Extreme fatigue, so often experienced by dying people, lowers perception levels and limits the time available for communications. When the day is punctuated with sleep episodes it is easy to lose track of events, everything becomes somewhat blurred. In times of exhaustion patients and their hard-pressed relatives need to be freed from the compulsion towards verbal communication and reassured that a comforting, quiet presence may convey the message of love as effectively.

It is not safe to assume levels of consciousness. Long after the patient has lost the ability to communicate he may be receptive to touch and hearing. Mary had appeared to be unconscious for several hours and had not in the past given any indication that she was aware of her condition. A visitor stood by her bed and said to a nurse, 'Poor thing, she hasn't long to go now, has she?' Immediately a stream of tears was seen to trickle from under Mary's closed eyelids. She died shortly after. It is so important that nurses are aware of this situation and that they convey this awareness to relatives. This knowledge can then be used to good rather than bad effect when the family are able to communicate comforting words.

There is much that nurses can do when the patient's condition makes communications difficult. They may first of all encourage with real interest and patience, employing all the senses. Then there are a variety of aids ranging from the simple picture chart to the electronic. Lastly, when the patient appears unconscious, gentle touch and simple cheerful words may be able to continue to bring comfort and support.

Emotional states

The days or weeks of terminal care are often ones of stress for the patient and his family when each is trying to come to terms with the situation. The family may be exhausted after trying to cope at home; a wife, for example, having to shoulder the care of her husband and his business responsibilities on top of her usual commitments. Even when the patient is in hospital the continual visiting is physically and emotionally tiring and disruptive of the daily routine.

In such times of stress various defence mechanisms and reactions emerge and these affect communication. Relatives may feel numb and appear to lack any emotion, they may become depressed, or they may become angry and direct their anger on to some aspect of care. Thus a presenting problem, generating much feeling, may be not enough sugar in a patient's cup of tea, but the real problem a deep anguish and sense of guilt about not being able to cope any longer with the loved one at home. Families are in a state of anticipated bereavement; they may be extra sensitive, or the anxiety that they suffer may prevent them from absorbing information. It is sometimes necessary to repeat explanations several times.

Patients who are becoming aware of their prognosis experience various emotional states which have been defined as denial, anger, bargaining, depression and acceptance. Feelings may vary with the appearance and disappearance of symptoms; so that successful control of symptoms can lead to denial once more of the true situation. There is therefore often no firm basis for a communication approach, and it is necessary to be constantly observant and perceptive.

A further complexity arises from the need to understand how best to offer help. Differences in personality and background provide diverse means of expression requiring different responses; thus the same degree of resentment might be felt by a little old lady and a young man but each would be likely to express it in a different way. One might prefer a silent empathy, the other encouragement to talk. Many people respond to gentle touch but not all. Sensitivity is needed to discern what is required.

It is not easy to cope in all circumstances and surely learning how to do so is a life-long task. When there are problems it does help if the various manifestations of feeling can be steadfastly and uncritically accepted by the nurse, who can offer a listening presence. The shared wisdom of the team can also be applied to meeting a need, and this will provide support to all concerned.

The social environment

It is not very often that the patient's needs for communication in human interaction can be entirely met by staff and personal visitors. Patients derive much comfort from each other and from each other's visitors. Here they depend upon the perception and willingness of nurses to place them near to compatible persons.

This is often far from easy in a hospital ward, where there may be frequent admissions and discharges of those not terminally ill, or in a special unit, where deaths occur when relationships have been made and there is always the possibility of being placed with someone who is unable to communicate. The effects can be far-reaching, for example an aphasic patient may become extremely depressed if he is placed for long periods next to one who is unconscious. He could benefit from watching others who are more active, communicating with them in non-verbal ways. Similarly one who needs to talk should not constantly accompany one who lacks this ability. Compatibility with others may also have much to do with personality and life experience as well as physical ability to communicate.

It would be unrealistic to think that communication systems may be tailored closely to the needs of each patient all the time. Frequent movement may have to be balanced against the needs for stability. However, there can be a continual awareness of social contact needs, and a review whenever there is change, with the goal of placing compatible persons together for at least part of each day.

Messages we seek to communicate to patients and their families

If we had to choose one word to describe the over-all content of messages to patients and their families, this could well be safety or security. We want them to know that even if cure is not possible they may feel safe in hands that are skilled to meet the needs of the present circumstances. We want them to understand that all our skills will be applied to the detection and treatment of symptoms and that through every emotional upheaval patients and their families will be accepted and supported as unique and valuable individuals. These safety messages must be clear and addressed to general and specific situations.

In general it is not easy to send clear messages even though attitudinal barriers have been overcome. There are many components of communication and clarity demands that they be in accord with one another. For example, a nurse might greet a patient, 'Good morning Mrs Brown. How are you today?' This enquiry may be perceived in different ways by Mrs Brown depending on how she is feeling and also on how the components of the message relate to each other. There are at least five important aspects of this communication apart from the words that are spoken; tone of voice, eye contact, proximity to Mrs Brown, bodily movement of the speaker and use of pause for reply.

Mrs Brown will be helped to confide her worries if she senses genuine concern behind the question and feels the nurse wants to give of her time. The nurse will best convey this attitude if there is interest in her tone of voice, if she engages in eye contact, stands close enough to the bed to encourage conversation, stills her bodily movements that would indicate she might be in a hurry, and pauses to allow Mrs Brown time to reply. It would perhaps be even more helpful if the nurse is able to sit either on or by the bed so that she is on the same level as her patient.

A patient who is aware that his condition is deteriorating is likely to have a number of specific fears, which are shared by the family on his behalf – 'Perhaps I am going to die – what will dying be like? Will I be able to bear pain and sickness? What if I should choke or end up being unable to swallow? Will there be help when I need it – suppose I should be helpless and there were to be a fire?'

Other fears relate to loss of role and acceptability. 'How will the family manage if I die? Suppose I have to depend on others for absolutely everything and lose all my dignity, how could I bear that? Will I become incontinent or smell or look horrible so that people will not want to be near me? Will I be on my own when I die? What has been the point of my life?' These are some of the concerns expressed by people who are dying, to which safety messages are addressed in a variety of different ways.

Communicating security through the environment

Even when one is in full health it can be frightening to meet with a strange environment. Patients who enter an institution for terminal care may have been fighting off admission for some time even though they are acutely uncomfortable. To consent to be admitted is to agree openly that things are not improving; it is to relinquish what may be seen as the last vestige of normality and to consider more fully that perhaps life is coming to an end. For the relatives, it may mean accepting that they no longer are fully able to cope, which often carries an undeserved feeling of guilt. The time of admission therefore is one of extreme sensitivity and first impressions are very important. The components of the security messages here are an attractive physical environment and a warm welcome.

A pleasing environment has much to say. A clean, bright building conveys the sense of good management, order and care through which the hidden areas such as the kitchens will be safe. Bright curtains and furnishings are cheering, and carefully tended flowers and plants are reminders of hope, love, and the natural world outside. They may speak to some of a Creator who cares for details. Carefully chosen pictures convey the feeling that here is a place that is aware of more than physical need. Last but not least, a smiling staff who look neat and attractive transmit the message of high morale and a happy atmosphere.

Security is also derived from a sense of belonging, of being drawn into the life of the ward. Patients are introduced to each other and told or shown the ward arrangements and details of the daily routine. They are greeted by name, and concern is shown for their belongings and for their individuality and personal tastes. The family will feel more secure if they know of expectations regarding visiting, where the visitor's lavatories are situated, where they may rest or have a snack or buy extras for the patient. Whenever possible, patients and their families are offered a tray of tea.

Attention to these small details has great value, not only because each is important in its own right, but because together they closely follow the pattern of Western social custom which denotes hospitality and acceptance in a variety of situations.

Communicating security through availability and awareness

One of the greatest supports to the patient and his family is the knowledge that someone is available to help when needed. The problem is that in a busy ward it is difficult to be available to everyone all the time. To some extent ward staffing levels rely on the fact that only a few needs will be presented at any one time. When this is not the case, nurses have to make good use of the factors that communicate interest and willingness to give attention as soon as possible.

Some relatives stood by the bedside of an elderly lady who had been knocked down by a car. It was thought that she might not live and because of her bad condition she had been placed near to the sister's desk. The sister was busy writing and did not look up or greet them. They wanted to speak to her but even though they approached the desk she still did not raise her eyes to show she was available. After an hour they sadly left not liking to disturb a professional person who seemed to be intent on some important task. They couldn't help feeling that they mattered so little; they also worried that staff might be too busy to cope if something suddenly went wrong with their mother. This sister might well have had a hectic day and have been under pressure to catch up on her administrative work, but a glance and smile would have been sufficient to indicate that she was aware of the family and would give her full attention when she could.

Whether we are passing visitors in the corridor or a patient who does not need us at present, it is so important to indicate that we are aware of their presence. To show awareness means to acknowledge the person, to communicate that they matter; it transmits empathy in a traumatic situation and gives patients and relatives good reason to feel that their needs will be readily observed. To express this awareness is of course no substitute for giving our whole attention to the patient when required, but when we are very pressurized it does enable people to wait for a short time secure in the knowledge that we both know and care about them.

Nurses are often afraid of the situation where an insecure patient makes constant demands on their attention and react with feigned unawareness and avoidance behaviour. This tends to make matters worse. We need to use the time spent on bedside nursing to offer our whole attention to patients so that through conversation and use of silence they may be encouraged to express their fears. They may well be helped towards calmness if they are sure of their means of communication, for example a bell placed at hand and secured so that it cannot slip. We may be able to enlist the help of volunteer helpers to sit with frightened patients, or organize visits from the family so that they are a little spread out. Our willingness to accept the patient's feelings indicates our ready involvement in the total situation, and if this is offered steadily and uncritically through all the manifestations of fear, anger and grief, then it communicates to the patient that as a unique person he is secure.

As the patient's life draws to a close our previous meaningful communication with him and his family may help us to perceive what he would like best. Many people are comforted by the presence of someone else, not necessarily a nurse, at this lonely time. This will bring security not only to the individual concerned but to other patients who will be watching. Another form of availability is to be prepared to support the patient according to his own cultural values and beliefs, so whatever our own ideas we must be ready, for example, to read a prayer or a passage from appropriate scriptures, or to find someone who will better be able to help. It is not easy to act in this way, especially at first, as our natural inhibitions and professional training have often taught us to deny such situations. It is, however, what true availability demands.

Communicating security through practical skills

Skilled nursing has great potential for communicating security at all levels. For example, the hot, sticky patient who has tossed around in bed is expertly washed and handled with gentle assurance. Lying in bed, cooler, and in a new position, she feels physically comforted and secure. But this is not where her comfort ends; the gentleness of the nurse and the personal interest she has taken have eased her general fears, particularly if she has been able to confide a little. The care the nurse has taken to preserve her privacy and to involve her in every possible decision – 'What nightdress would you like today – how many pillows?' – has boosted her dignity and made her feel a little more like a real person. Lastly, the attention the nurse has given to replacing her things on the locker as she will require them has indicated that her needs are anticipated. She then has reason to believe that should she become helpless and inarticulate she will be in safe hands. What a lot of security is obtained from the 'ordinary' task.

Communicating security through systematic observation and enquiry
Perhaps one of the greatest boosts to a patient's sagging morale is to experience relief from some long-standing symptom such as pain. It can bring the feeling that despite everything life is still worth living. This type of relief often results from the close observation and attention to detail of each member of the care team, who will enquire regularly about the patient's state.

Of itself this enquiry will bring the patient a sense of safety, especially if it is made clear that small details are important. Patients so often feel they should not bother busy staff with items they see as trivial. The nurse may also use a planned Nursing Process type assessment to give breadth as well as depth to her enquiry, and her systematic approach will be another source of confidence for the patient. Her findings will assist other members of the team in their own forms of enquiry.

When the combined approach of the team brings symptom control in one area, then the patient is encouraged to trust for the future despite his fears and to feel secure in safe hands.

Communicating security through offering 'the extra'
We all have expectations of a variety of situations in life, and these are based on our attitudes and the values we have absorbed from society. We therefore accept certain standards of behaviour as normal and are aggrieved when they are not met rather than appreciative when they are. When something happens that is above our expectations, then this has an impact.

This something extra may be the means through which a breakthrough in trusting relationships is achieved. For example, patients arriving at some units are met and welcomed by a very senior member of staff. This really emphasizes to the patient his importance as an individual and the concern that is felt for him. Much depends upon the possibilities within each institutional setting; many such extras cannot be planned in advance but are imaginative personal responses to the needs of the time.

Thus one nurse may go to great lengths to find something special for her patient to eat, the ward staff may combine to plan a celebration of a patient's birthday or relax their own ideas of ward arrangement to meet the differing expectations of someone from a different cultural background. Another member of staff may show interest and respect for the patient in taking time to learn from him or to facilitate his participation in a hobby. An exhausted relative whose numb feelings make him feel guilty and callous may be surprised to meet with real sympathy and understanding.

The point is that the patient's expectations rather than the nurse's ideals are exceeded, and a perceptive nurse may find many occasions in which she can bring surprise and pleasure to him. When circumstances make it very hard to trust it is these kinds of 'extras' that help lift the fear.

Conclusion

Meaningful communication with the patient, the family, and with other members of the health care team is the basis of effective terminal care. Many hazards can be encountered, not least the attitudes and expectations of all concerned. These need to be honestly identified. Once this has been accomplished safety messages may be sent. If they are to be clearly received, their components must be skilfully blended to form a united picture. This choosing and blending process has potential for great reward – the comforting of body and mind of the patient and his family, and perhaps some achievement of a goal that is special to him. This presents an exciting challenge that must be met with both the science and art of nursing.

References

Argyl, M (1973) Social Interaction, Tavistock

Browning, M E and Lewis, E P (1972) The dying patient: a nursing perspective, American Journal of Nursing

Folta, J R (1965) The perception of death, Nursing Research, 14, Summer

Harper, B (1977) Death: The Coping Mechanism of the Health Professional, Southeastern University Press, Greenville, S C

Hurst, S (1977) Shaken By The Wind, Mayhew-McCrimmon Ltd, Great Wakering, Essex. (A patient's experiences in verse)

Koff, H (1980) Hospice – A caring community, Winthrop

Kubler-Ross, E (1970) On Death and Dying, Tavistock

Parkes, C Murray (1972) Bereavement, Pelican Books

Reynolds, D K and Kalish, R A (1974) The social ecology of dying: observations of wards of the terminally ill, Hospital and Community Psychiatry, 25, March

Saunders, C M, Summers, D and Teller, N (eds) (1981) Hospice: the living idea, Edward Arnold

Shusterman, L R (1973) Death and dying: a critical review of literature, Nursing Outlook, 21 July

Smith, B (1965) Dear Gift of Life: A man's encounter with death, Pendle Hill Pamphlet 142, USA

West, T S and Kirkham, S R (1981) The Family, in Saunders et al. (Editors) Hospice: the living idea, Edward Arnold

CHAPTER 8

CARE DURING THE LAST HOURS OF LIFE
SISTER MARCELLA CASSELLS and K M PFISTER

Signs of approaching death

It is important to remember that, as always, patients during their last hours are individuals and each one will react in his or her own way – and that trying to assess what are in fact the last hours may not be easy, even for experienced nurses. There are many occasions when the nurse concerned is convinced that the patient will die before morning, but, to her amazement, he survives for several more days.

Some terminally ill patients die suddenly from severe haemorrhage, a pulmonary embolus or coronary thrombosis, but the great majority gradually get weaker as their vital functions become less able to cope, and many then pass gently into unconsciousness and finally into respiratory or cardiac failure.

Changes nurses may observe in terminally ill patients

Nurses who are attending the patient throughout the 24 hours are often the first to observe changes which indicate impending death. These may be summarized as follows:

1   There may be a gradual loss of interest in what is happening round them – social disengagement – but this is not universal, and many patients retain their interest in life to the very end.

2   Patients whose symptoms have so far been well controlled may become restless, agitated and obviously uncomfortable. They may start plucking at the bedclothes and a slight frown or tautness of the facial muscles may indicate the presence of underlying pain or discomfort. General weakness or drowsiness may prevent the patient from describing his complaint. As actual pain may be present, even if the patient is in coma, analgesics should not be withdrawn, but they may sometimes be reduced.

3   They become increasingly unwilling or unable to take food or fluids. The mouth is usually very dry, as these patients frequently breathe through the mouth.

4   Changes in colour may occur: extreme pallor; cyanosis; jaundice. In these days when we live in a multi-racial society, it is essential to learn to observe the differences in colour which take place in those with black, brown or yellow skins.

5   Changes in pulse rate and rhythm are important observations. The pulse may become weak, thready, rapid and irregular – it may no longer be felt at the wrist, but have to be taken at the carotid artery in the neck, or it may be necessary to feel for the heartbeat. With the hand held over the apex of the heart one can actually feel the heartbeat stop completely; quite a dramatic moment.

6   Changes in breathing are often a sign of impending death and can take various forms. Stridulous or noisy breathing, sometimes called the death rattle, is due to the accumulation of secretions in the larynx and trachea which the patient is too weak to cough up. Air hunger – gasping for air – may be associated with internal haemorrhage and is also a very distressing sign. Cheyne-Stokes respirations involve periods of apnoea, followed by increasingly rapid respirations which reach a peak and then gradually become quieter till apnoea occurs again. This cycle is often repeated until breathing ceases for good. The jaw may droop or be tightly clenched. Uraemia may cause foetor and/or hiccups.

7   The eyes may be staring, squinting or have a rather glazed look, and in wasting diseases, where the fatty pads lining the eyeballs has dissolved, there is a hollow-eyed appearance which is very characteristic. Sometimes the eyes are closed, or they may remain open even when the patient is unconscious; a somewhat eerie effect. Occasionally, the eyes may be positively fixed on some object apparently visible to the patient but not seen by others.

8   Due to the relaxation of the sphincter muscles, incontinence of urine and/or faeces may occur; though at times retention and faecal impaction are present and give rise to restlessness.

9   Increasing coldness of the body can be observed, especially obvious in the limbs, and cold sweat often appears on the face and hands.

10   Altered states of consciousness are common: the patient may fail to respond to stimuli, then appear to regain some degree of response – twitchings may occur – then eventually there is a lapse into the coma preceding death. There is often a noticeable change in expression: after an almost agonized look, the calm, peace and serenity of death may be very striking. The patient may also appear younger than in life as after a while lines disappear from the face and a youthful smoothness is seen. In *Henry V*, Shakespeare gives a truly graphic description of the signs of approaching death when Mistress Quickly tells of Falstaff's last hours: ' 'a parted ev'n just between twelve and one, ev'n at the turning o' th' tide: for after I saw him fumble with the sheets, and play with flowers, and smile upon his finger's end, I knew there was but one way; for his nose was as sharp as a pen, and 'a babbled of green fields.'

Nursing care of patients during the last hours of life

This care will make all the difference to the dying patient and must be carried out with great gentleness and understanding.

As the patient's general condition becomes steadily weaker, the drugs given to control pain continue to be given, as ordered by the doctor. Sometimes the dose is reduced, particularly if renal failure is apparent, and the drugs are best given as suppositories or by injection. If bronchial secretions are causing a problem, drugs such as hyoscine, atropine and frusemide may be prescribed to help relieve this. Suction may also be used to clear the air passages of secretions, but this may cause some distress to the patient and it must be done with extreme gentleness and skill.

All usual nursing care is given to ensure that the patient is kept clean, dry and as comfortable as possible. It is important to change the patient's position regularly, especially if he appears to be lying awkwardly, and every effort must be made to place him where he is able to breathe most easily and is not putting pressure on any sore he may have. Skilful arrangement of pillows and support for the feet may make all the difference to his comfort and this may need to be repeated at frequent intervals if he is inclined to be restless. A bed cradle may help to relieve pressure from bed-clothes. Gowns which are loose and open easily for treatment to be carried out are convenient and cause less disturbance to the patient, and a light shawl or bedjacket to protect the shoulders is useful, especially if the patient is in a propped-up position. Careful sponging-down may be given instead of a bed-bath, which may be somewhat exhausting for the patient. A compress wrung out of cool water or eau de cologne and placed on the forehead often relieves headache and may be found soothing and refreshing. Care of the pressure areas is continued without too much disturbance and any actual sores or other wounds are treated as necessary. If there is an unpleasant odour due to a discharging wound, a deodorant spray may be useful. The importance of keeping bed linen clean and fresh and of making sure that the patient is comfortably warm, but not overheated cannot be stressed too strongly. A bed is the patient's last home, so to speak, and must be made in such a way as to provide the maximum rest and comfort for the occupant.

As many patients at this stage breathe through the mouth and are often reluctant to drink, the care of the mouth is of the utmost importance. A dry mouth adds greatly to the patient's discomfort, so regular attention to the mouth is necessary: glycerine of thymol may be used on foam stick applicators and a soothing cream applied to the lips, especially if they are beginning to crack. This treatment must be carried out with great care as the patient frequently resists it. Dentures must be removed if the patient is semiconscious. If there are no sores or cracks in the mouth or lips, a small piece of lemon can be given to the patient to suck and is both cleansing and refreshing.

Other methods include giving the patient chopped ice, flavoured according to his taste, or sweets to suck – or pineapple to chew – or a moisturizing drink (artificial saliva may be used consisting of methylcellulose with a flavouring of orange or lemon – make 1 g up to 100 ml with water and give small sips frequently).

Care of the eyes is also essential, especially if they remain open: bathing with normal saline lotion or hypromellose (artificial tears), instilling soothing eye drops and occasionally placing soft eye pads over the lids in the case of unconscious patients whose eyes remain open. This may upset the patient's relatives if they are visiting and a full explanation of why this treatment is being carried out should be given to them.

If the patient is suffering from retention of urine or is incontinent, a self-retaining catheter is passed and drains into a bag. This is changed as required and the amount and colour of the urine is noted.

Faecal impaction may be present and may account for restlessness. If the doctor agrees, measures can be taken to relieve this, or it may be considered best not to disturb the patient at this stage, but to try and relieve the restlessness by giving appropriate drugs, e.g. diazepam or chlorpromazine.

Throughout these last hours, the nurse's approach to the dying person must be one of care, support and sympathetic understanding. Some patients are in great fear and dread of death and have not come to terms with their illness. They are in urgent need of spiritual help even if they themselves are not aware of this. They should never be left alone when their condition has deteriorated and death is expected soon. A relative, friend or the nurse should be at the bedside and available to comfort and support the patient. One cannot stress too strongly the value of touch, which keeps the dying person in contact with those around him: holding his hand, gently caressing his back and talking to him quietly all help him in his last moments. One must always remember that hearing is the last sense that is lost and often the patient can hear someone speaking even if he is apparently in coma. The nurse should never say anything in the presence of the seemingly unconscious patient which would not be said to his face.

If the relatives are present, they are asked if they would like suitable prayers to be said at the bedside. These may be led by a chaplain of the appropriate denomination, by the ward sister or staff nurse, and the relatives are usually eager to participate.

We must remember that many of our patients belong to religious faiths which are not Christian and that they may have strong views on how they should be treated and cared for at the hour of death. These views must always be scrupulously respected and if a minister of their own faith is available he should be sent for in good time. Nurses should take the trouble to inform themselves regarding the religious and cultural background of their patients, so as to be able to give the maximum help and support at this critical time.

Nurses who have not been present at a death before may feel rather nervous and anxious at such a time, and a senior nurse should do all that is possible to help them understand their feelings and to realize that death comes to us all – that it is a fact we must learn to live with. It should be stressed that by acting in a positive manner with the dying patient one can help him to overcome the natural fear of death.

Care of the relatives

Looking after the dying patient's family and close friends is often a delicate problem requiring great tact and skill. They may have feelings of guilt or resentment, may be apathetic or aggressive, deeply concerned or apparently uninterested. At such times one sees not only the best in human nature but, unfortunately, also the worst. Some relatives seem to be interested only in any money or belongings of the patient which they think are theirs by rights. One should try not to judge others and learn to adapt to the changing moods shown by the family. It should always be remembered that some of them may have been under great stress and strain – emotional, financial, spiritual – for some time, and allowances should be made for what may appear to be callous behaviour but may instead be their way of hiding their true feelings.

Here again we must bear in mind the cultural background which may affect the relatives' behaviour: from the severely stoical, 'stiff upper-lip' attitude to the highly emotional ways of displaying grief.

The patient who is admitted to an institution

As a patient may be admitted at a very late stage for terminal care, the following paragraphs offer some guidelines in dealing with relatives. The relatives should be seen by the doctor and ward sister and a simple but clear explanation of the patient's condition and likely prognosis given to them. They should have the opportunity to ask questions and told that they will always be welcome to visit at any time convenient to them and to stay if wished during the night. If they can in any way help with the care of the patient, e.g. by moistening the lips, they should be encouraged to do so. A telephone number where the next of kin can be reached in an emergency is helpful, or failing that the telephone number of a nearby friend or the police station nearest the home. Enquiries regarding the religious faith of the patient should be made and any special requests for a minister to be sent for should be carefully noted. For example, in the case of a Jewish patient, the name, address and telephone number of the Rabbi or his deputy must be available with the patient's case notes, and the family's wishes regarding Last Offices ascertained.

Relatives must be gently informed of the deterioration in the patient's condition and of the changes which can be expected during the following day or hours. If it is their wish to be present when the patient dies, the nurse must make sure she knows how to contact them. Some relatives, on the other hand, do not wish to be at the bedside of the dying person and it is not for the nurse to judge these people unfavourably. They may not wish to break down before others or have reasons which are not obvious for their actions.

All relatives must be reassured that the dying person is kept free from pain and is as comfortable as possible under the circumstances. They should be reminded that even an apparently unconscious patient may be able to hear what they say. The importance of touch must also be stressed: holding the patient's hand and giving it a reassuring squeeze gives the dying patient the sense that he is not alone.

When death seems imminent, depending on the faith of the patient, prayers can be said by the appropriate minister of religion or a member of staff. These prayers should be very simple and said very slowly and clearly.

Exactly what to say or do at such times will depend on so many different circumstances that no hard and fast rules can be laid down. One must react as one thinks best and give support and sympathy to the family at this critical moment.

In recognizing the signs of death, the nurse will observe the cessation of respiration and of the heartbeat (which may sometimes be present even after no pulse can be felt in the wrist). This indicates that these vital functions of the body are no longer present. However, it must be noted that at the present time this definition of death is inadequate; a patient who has had a cardiac arrest will have no pulse nor be breathing but may still be alive and able to be resuscitated. Likewise, a patient attached to a ventilator may be dead although his respirations are being maintained. Further discussion of this problem of legal definition of death will be found in Chapter 16.

When a patient has died the nurse has a duty to inform the doctor who has been treating the patient, as he is the only person who can certify the death. Although he must have seen the deceased prior to death there is no legal requirement that he must view the body after death. Circumstances will dictate whether the doctor is sent for immediately, e.g. in the case of sudden or unexpected death, or whether he is informed later.

As soon as the patient has died, the nurse must be ready to deal with a variety of reactions. The family should be allowed to remain with the deceased for a short while, then offered the privacy of a room where they can, if they wish to, be alone, or, if they prefer it, pour out their emotions to a sympathetic listener. A tray of tea is of great value in many cases and helps people to calm down and become less tense. It is essential to explain to the bereaved that it is perfectly natural in such circumstances to cry and be upset: it is part of the pattern of bereavement and is to be expected. Some relatives may experience feelings of guilt or relief from strain, and may act in totally unpredictable ways which may be somewhat disturbing. The nurse should not appear to be upset by this, but allow the individuals to get rid of their tensions in any way they like and just be there to offer help.

Sometimes the nurse herself may be particularly moved by the patient's death, and share in the grief of the relatives in a spontaneous expression of emotion such as putting her arms round a relative and shedding a few tears. This demonstration of closeness is often very comforting to the family, but naturally this must be combined with the nurse continuing in her role of supporter in a calm and capable manner. There may also be less experienced young colleagues who need her example and help in coping with their own emotions whilst caring for the family.

If any social problems are likely to occur as a result of the death, the relatives will have been referred to the social worker, who will be able to give help and advice. If additional support is necessary, as in the case of a father left with young children or an elderly person left without relatives, a Bereavement Team is valuable to visit regularly and use their skills to assist in every way possible. The team may consist of trained volunteers.

Last Offices

Once again the religion and cultural background of the dead person must be considered and care taken not to offend the beliefs of the family by thoughtless actions.

In the case of Christians or those of no particular faith the body is washed, any catheters or other appliances removed, and any sores or wounds covered with a simple dressing; body orifices may be packed and the lower jaw supported with a bandage. Dentures, if worn, are usually left in, but it is best to get the consent of the relatives regarding this and also regarding any rings or other jewellery worn by the patient. One is sometimes surprised to find that the family, perhaps for financial reasons, wish to keep the jewellery and even the false teeth. The body may be taken to a Chapel of Rest where the relatives can see it before the undertakers remove it.

In the case of other faiths, the exact action to be taken after death must be ascertained and strictly adhered to. Orthodox Jews do not wish the body to be handled by non-Jews, and the same applies to Moslems and Hindus. It is sad enough for the family to have lost a loved one without adding to their distress by doing something abhorrent to them.

Legal aspects

Nurses need to know the principles of the legal aspects involved just before and after the death of a patient. They may be asked questions by the relatives and should be able to answer them.

Next of kin   It is very important to establish who is the next of kin and where he/she may be contacted. One would think this was an easy task, but it is not always so, as one discovers through bitter experience; for example two ladies may claim to be the wife of the patient or a hitherto unknown relative may turn up and insist he is the next of kin. Much tact is needed to deal with such situations.

Time of death   The exact time of death should be noted and the doctor, if not present, should be informed (see p. 107).

Who was present at the time of death?   The names of those present are recorded: relatives and staff.

Last Offices   As already mentioned in the section on Last Offices, the relatives' wishes must be ascertained, to avoid possible future litigation as well as natural distress. If there is any question of criminal proceedings there should be minimal interference with the body.

Question of a post-mortem   If the cause of death is uncertain a post-mortem may be necessary and this must be carefully explained to the next of kin, as the coroner will have to be informed. Even if the cause of death is clear, the doctor may wish to carry out a post-mortem, and for this he must obtain the consent of the nearest relative.

Property of the deceased patient   Any valuables or large sums of money should already have been deposited for safe keeping with the hospital administrator, and the nearest relative can collect them when convenient. Other belongings usually kept in the bedside locker should be listed by two nurses who then sign the list as a correct record. The property is packed into a parcel or box and may be given to the relatives at a suitable moment, usually when they come for the death certificate.

Existence of a valid will   Nurses may be questioned regarding the advisability of making a will and should encourage all patients who are terminally ill to make one, as this prevents much friction and even family feuds after the death. If, however, they are asked to act as witnesses to a patient's will, they are well advised not to do so, but to suggest that a solicitor should see the patient and find witnesses. As a valuable document, the will can then be deposited for safe keeping with the hospital administrator, if this is what the patient desires.

Death certificates   If the cause of death is clear, the doctor caring for the patient will sign the death certificate, and arrangements can be made for the relative to collect this and take it to the registrar as soon as possible. If there are any doubtful circumstances, the doctor will report the death to the coroner and the certificate will be marked to this effect.

Identification of the dead person in hospital   It is very important to avoid mistakes, and preferably the body should be clearly labelled, for instance by leaving the identity bracelet in place. It is insufficient to mark only the outside of the shroud.

Donation of organs for transplant or of the whole body for medical research   The nearest relative must act quickly if it was the wish of the dead person to donate organs for transplant or the body for research: kidneys must be removed within half an hour of death and eyes within 6 hours, so there is no time to be lost if the donor's wishes are to be complied with. The nurse's involvement with this matter will consist in making sure that the relatives are in touch with the doctor concerned, and in being aware that, as with a request for a post-mortem or coroner's inquest examination, this can add to distress and increase the need for support at this time.

Cremation   The law requires a further certificate signed by two doctors (one if a post-mortem is to take place) before cremation can be carried out.

Sudden and unexpected death

The family of a person who dies quite unexpectedly, having been last seen apparently fit and well, are likely to pass through a series of severe reactions. At first there will be bewilderment and failure to comprehend what has happened, followed by a state of shock. The deceased person may have been found dead at home, or brought to a hospital already dead.

The relatives will need treating with gentleness and compassion and should not be left alone. A friend or less involved member of the family who can give warm but calm support will be a great asset to the nurse in her efforts to support the relatives at this initial stage. There may be uncontrollable crying, or a feeling of numbness and unreality. Later, the relatives will want to talk about the situation with doctor and nurse, and ask questions about the circumstances of the death. They are likely to ask to see the body, and should be prepared for any possibly distressing features.

One of the most tragic situations is if the deceased person has committed suicide, without any apparent intimation of this. Inevitably the family will question whether they are to blame and could have done anything to avert the tragedy. They will need to talk about their feelings, and their deceased relative, and may need long-term professional support during the process of mourning. In all these distressing situations, careful explanation must be given in simple terms and in an unhurried way.

References

Hanratty, J F (1981) Control of Distressing Symptoms in the Dying Patient, St Joseph's Hospice

Hanratty, J F (1983) Care of the Dying – Philosophy of the care of terminal illness, St Joseph's Hospice

Sampson, C (1982) The Neglected Ethic – Religious and cultural factors in the care of patients, McGraw-Hill

Young, A P (1981) Legal Problems in Nursing Practice, Harper and Row

CHAPTER 9

CARE IN THE HOME
HARRIET COPPERMAN

Introduction

The industrialized, affluent parts of the world have, comparatively recently, seen a gradual move towards death occurring in a hospital or other institution rather than dying people remaining in their own homes. In Britain and the United States of America 60–70% of deaths now occur in a hospital (Simpson 1979).

There are several reasons for this. Families are smaller than previously so that greater strain is placed on the carers. The unmarried members of the family often do not stay under the same roof but move off to a separate existence elsewhere. Many mothers now go out to work so that a dying relative would be alone much of the day anyway. Today there is much more population movement than hitherto, so that often families live in different towns or parts of the country, and may even have emigrated.

Another possible reason for people not dying at home is fear in the care givers. Over the last half century, because of dramatic reductions in the likelihood of death in infancy, childhood and young adulthood, many people reach middle age and have still never seen anyone dead or dying – especially as there has not been a major war for nearly 40 years.

Thus, when presented with a dying person many families will panic, feel inadequate and urge admission for their loved one.

Advantages of home care

What of that loved one – where does he want to die? Given the opportunity, most people would like to die in their own home and their own bed. One of the most traumatic experiences in life must be to have an ambulance drawing up at the door to take a very ill person to hospital. For that individual knows – even if he hasn't verbalized it – that he is seeing his home of perhaps 40 years or more for the last time. The garden so lovingly tended and the tomato plants about to flower will not be seen again. The dog who leapt on the bed every morning to waken his master will not be seen again, as animals are not usually allowed into hospitals. Finally, the bed warmly shared with a spouse for the past 40 years will never be experienced again either. So much to lose at a time of life when such things could bring the greatest comfort to the dying. So, with a determined nurse and other members of the primary care team the aim should be to enable the death to take place at home. Domiciliary hospice teams around the country and the world have shown that the trend towards dying in an 'institution' is reversible. Many of these teams report 60–80% of their patients dying at home.

Thus admission should be for social reasons only, for instance an elderly and infirm spouse, or an elderly patient living alone. Medical and nursing problems can usually be resolved in the home – apart from a few occasions when a patient or family finds it difficult to co-operate for whatever reason. There are many differences between caring for a dying patient at home and doing so in hospital. Noticeable are the role reversals. The patient and his family are the hosts and the nurse or doctor is the visitor.

In hospital it is usually possible to 'persuade' a patient to do things he doesn't like, for instance taking multifarious pleasant or unpleasant medications and treatments. At home the patient is king of his domain; not a frightened man in bed with a label on his wrist to distinguish him from his neighbour. He can show the nurse the door if he does not like her approach or what she is offering.

Another difference is that in a hospital setting, although relatives are treated with polite courtesy, they might be regarded as a bit of a nuisance – they clutter up and untidy the ward, they often want to be talked with and ask awkward questions, and they are always bringing flowers which have to be put in water and which get knocked over when the curtains are pulled round the bed!

At home the patient and family are considered to be one unit requiring care. Many times the relatives need as much if not more help than the patient.

Assessment

With practice this should become continuous and almost subconscious. It begins before meeting the patient. What sort of area is the home in? Does the outside look cared for or neglected? What do the curtains at the windows look like: ragged and dirty or immaculate – or somewhere in between? What sounds are there before the door opens – arguing and raised voices, dogs and screaming children, or nothing? Consider the state of the person opening the door – do the eyes look away, look anxious or frightened or weary, or bright and happy and welcoming? Is the home well cared for and well loved, or is it a cold, sad, lonely home? Is the neglect long-term or due to the illness of the patient? Note the arrangement of furniture – chairs in isolated positions may indicate the nature of the occupants.

The emotional state of the people in the home needs assessing: for example, is the spouse defensive or nervous or over-protective? The patient's manner of greeting and subsequent conversation should reveal whether he is angry, anxious, depressed, terrified, happy, dull, unintelligent, unkempt, in pain, restless, agitated or confused.

Conversation with the patient and family and examination of the patient should also reveal all that is relevant in relation to nausea, vomiting, pain, bowels, bladder, mouth, sleep, cough, pressure areas, mobility, oedema, dyspnoea, wounds, discharges, bleeding and appetite.

All of these aspects should be assessed by the nurse (and the general practitioner will make his own assessment). The findings need to be accurately recorded. Nursing notes in the patient's home should, however, contain only information which would not alarm or upset the patient or family if read by them. Such matters as the degree of acceptance or denial of the diagnosis would have to be recorded at the health centre or wherever the more formal notes are stored. The patient's insight should be assessed but without probing too deeply. Asking the patient what he had radiotherapy for will often give a pointer to his degree of insight. On a first meeting, that is probably as far as the questioning should go in relation to diagnosis and prognosis – unless the patient is obviously wanting to discuss these matters further. At the first meeting it is also useful to enquire discreetly about the patient's religious faith, and how meaningful it is to him. The nurse will then have an idea as to whether or how the clergy should be involved later on. Throughout the patient's illness, communication is a vital aspect of care. This has been developed in Chapter 7.

Care of the family

The degree of effective help and support given to the family can make the difference between their coping or not coping. If they cannot cope, then the patient will usually have to leave his home and be admitted to hospital. This will often mean that a spouse will feel guilty and the subsequent bereavement will be more painful. The family have the rest of their lives to live after the death, and a distressing death and difficult bereavement period could drastically affect those lives, especially that of the spouse.

Often in families there is sibling rivalry, or one child may do most of the caring while the others feel guilty and become even less supportive. Thus, when the patient's needs have been met, the nurse often finds herself having a 15-minute 'doorstep chat' or else is spirited into the kitchen. She can then start to pick at and unravel some of the knots in the family, and allay some of their fears.

As mentioned earlier, fear of death is often why families do not cope. It is necessary to ascertain the nature of the fears. It can be difficult for a nurse to appreciate the incredible ideas held by the public about death. It is often thought to be explosive at the end, with guts spilling out and 'things' coming from the mouth. There is an idea that cancer creeps up in the throat – especially if the patient has a bronchial carcinoma – and strangles the patient so that he will choke. Another idea is that the patient will die screaming and in agony. With inadequate control of pain and other symptoms this does, unfortunately, happen.

Reassure the family that someone will always be available, even if only to answer a question on the telephone.

Reassure them that the patient will be given the best possible care and will probably die peacefully in his sleep – so peacefully that they may not realize immediately that he has died.

Check on the amount of sleep, food and recreation that the main care giver is having. Often there are many visitors and the spouse spends all day making tea and sandwiches. Offer to answer any questions they have.

Reassure them that the patient will not be 'told' anything he does not wish to hear. Teach the family whatever nursing techniques they want to do or are capable of doing. It is imperative not to increase their anxiety by asking them to perform tasks such as giving suppositories if such things frighten them. It is important to remember to praise the efforts of the family and to encourage them.

Some spouses will deny the impending death – their bereavement is likely to be difficult. Others will feel guilty about many things. If it relates to the care, the spouse should be reassured that the best nurse possible is the one who has known the patient for 40 years and knows exactly how he likes his tea made, and that without her he would have to be in hospital.

Relatives often ask for a prognosis because of taking time off from work. Although very tempting it is usually unwise to predict such matters. Very few babies (unless induced) are born on the expected day and few of us die when expected. A time limit can in fact cause more problems and anxiety for the family when death is quicker or slower than anticipated. It would be more useful, with the relative's agreement, to write a note to his/her employers, for example thanking them for being so helpful and understanding in allowing Mrs X time off to care for her very ill mother!

Another way to make life easier for the relatives is to deliver most of the medication so they do not have to keep queuing up at the doctor's surgery or the chemist. If there is time, allow them to go to the shops while nursing care is being given to the patient. Encouraging the relatives to cope when they feel they cannot is a decision which needs to be skilfully assessed. At the time the family may feel too much has been asked of them, but after the death they are usually pleased and delighted to find that they could manage. However, such pressure does require careful evaluation before being applied – some people cannot cope and should not be pushed too far.

The needs of children

Children in the family need care and often it is necessary to talk about it with the adults first. There is a tendency to hide children away from death in case it has some bad effect on them. The opposite is true. If, when someone has died, people behave as though there is something in the room so awful that a child cannot see it, he will grow up believing that death is too terrifying to behold. Children acquire attitudes from adults. It is easy to ask a child if he would like to say goodbye to

Grandma. He can be taken into the room and asked if he would like to kiss her goodbye. It is important to remember that an explanation of the death in adult terms may be misinterpreted by a child and produce undue anxiety. Obviously each child will have individual needs.

Children should be included in the grieving and not made to feel outsiders. There is usually no reason why they should not attend the funeral. There may be particular problems for the children when a parent dies. Can the other parent cope? This needs to be anticipated well before the death. The help of a social worker is likely to be necessary.

Care of the patient

The room or environment is of paramount importance. The situation is often improved if the living room is used as a bedroom. The advantages are that the patient remains in the circle of the family and is not isolated upstairs. It also saves the care giver from constantly going up and down stairs to attend to the patient's needs, and makes supervision much easier with less anxiety. Such a rearrangement should only be effected if all parties agree. Even if they are not going to move the patient's room, it may, with permission, be useful to move some of the furniture in the room to allow easier access to the patient.

The nurse needs to have frequent contact with the family by phone or visit. The aim is to anticipate needs rather than deal with a problem once it has arisen. The latter simply increases the family's anxiety, reducing the chance of keeping the patient at home. As the illness progresses new symptoms can and do present fairly frequently. The nurse needs to be aware of them in order to alert the doctor. The general practitioner should be given regular information and he can be kept on his toes by the nurse, for example, diagnosing oral thrush (very common in the dying) and suggesting nystatin drops for it! The number of visits by the nurse should increase as the patient deteriorates.

Medication, if prescribed confusingly at different times, will either be taken randomly or not at all. It is a good idea to request the doctor to prescribe so that drugs can be fitted easily into a 4, 8 or 12-hourly regime. Writing the medication out clearly will also increase the likelihood of accurate administration.

Equipment

Equipment for the dying patient needs to be provided sooner rather than later – later is likely to be too late. Ripple mattresses (large cell) can be very helpful for prevention of pressure sores. Bed cradle, bed, commode, urinal, feeding cup, bedpan, incontinence pad and sheeting, Zimmer frame and wheelchair may be needed and are usually available through local authorities.

Remember that in a patient's home there is no linen cupboard with an inexhaustible supply – only a tired family frantically borrowing from neighbours. Therefore incontinence needs to be anticipated so that a mattress is not ruined. An ideal draw mackintosh is made by cutting a black polythene bag (which most homes now have) down one long side and across the bottom. This can be put under the bottom sheet or draw sheet. Draw sheets can be manufactured by dissecting an old sheet. Families will often urge the nurse to cut up their best linen.

When a patient is dying, much of the management of the urinary tract can be initiated and carried out by the nurse (with the prior agreement of the doctor). Thus, if a semiconscious patient is incontinent or has an obvious retention with overflow, the natural thing will be to catheterize the patient without having to waste the precious time and comfort of the patient by obtaining equipment or trying to contact the doctor who may be out on his rounds. Condom drainage for male patients may be helpful if there is no retention.

Similarly, management of the bowel should be readily available. To have to wait another day or so in order to obtain suppositories simply prolongs the patient's discomfort while constipation turns into a faecal impaction. Should there be circumstances where a nurse could not catheterize or give immediate bowel care to a dying patient, then a plan should be made before the need arises. For example, a patient with carcinoma of the bladder may need to be hospitalized if a catheter is required, in case of acute haemorrhage.

The provision of equipment such as a commode may need tact and understanding. It is hard to recognize that the body one has taken for granted for so many years now no longer works properly. Patients may need to find out for themselves that they are unable to get to the toilet, before accepting a commode or urinal.

When a patient is dying at home, the week or so before unconsciousness develops can be difficult for him and the family. The patient gets cross at his weakness and inability and may displace his anger onto his family. This may increase their anguish. However, as the patient loses consciousness and begins to let go, the family's anxieties may become easier. This may also be because the nursing visits will have increased. A wife may be able to wash her conscious husband, but once he is unable to move himself the sensitive skill of a nurse may be needed to make the patient refreshed and comfortable. The frequency of 'turning' a patient at home may depend on how much the family can do, or the amount of domiciliary nursing available. The patient will need to be turned even in his own soft bed not less than 8-hourly. Relatives can be taught how to use foamstick applicators for clearing the mouth, and also how to give sips of water or medicine from them. The patient by this time does not care if he is not shaved, but the family's morale is lifted if his appearance is as normal as possible. A battery-operated razor is a useful piece of equipment in the nurse's bag.

An unconscious patient's medication needs to continue. Usually an 8-hourly regime can be organized in the home. Methadone (Physeptone) injection can be used but oxycodone suppositories are preferable to injections provided the opiate dose required is not more than 60 mg morphine (oral dose). One oxycodone suppository is equivalent to 30 mg morphine by mouth. The advantages are:

1   It is effective for 8 hours.
2   It causes less discomfort for the patient.
3   A relative may be able to insert it, thus reducing the number of nursing visits required.

If sedation is needed for restless patients, chlorpromazine (Largactil) suppositories 100 mg may be used. If injecting methadone, then methotrimiprazine 25–50 mg (as Nozinan) may be given with the same syringe. (Methotrimiprazine has greater strength and is in less volume than chlorpromazine in equivalent injection.)

Nurses are conditioned to sit patients up to prevent chest infections. Many patients dying of carcinomatosis and pneumonia are much more comfortable on their side with pillows giving plenty of support in the back, between neck and shoulder and between the knees. Nothing looks more distressing to a family than a patient lolling around either upright or semi-upright in bed.

After the death

After the patient has died and the family have been comforted, the body needs to be attended to. The nurse should be guided by the family, but in most instances it is not appropriate to do the full Last Offices as the undertaker can do these much more professionally. However, it is necessary in a home situation to remove catheters, straighten and tidy the body, insert dentures and support the jaw. The last is very simply done by wedging an appropriate-sized article between the chin and claviculo-sternal notch. A small perfume bottle or new bar of soap is often just right. The head should be on one or two pillows so that the sheet can be pulled just over the chin. The family can then be escorted in to say good-bye if they so wish. They often appreciate it if the nurse offers to contact the undertakers for them, who may collect the body straight away or wait until the doctor has issued the death certificate. Naturally, the general practitioner should be informed of the death. The nurse should ensure that a doctor has seen the patient not less than 2 weeks before the death in order to avoid unnecessary complications with legal requirements. Thus, for a patient dying at home, anticipation is the key to care. The other aim is maximum effectiveness with minimum fuss!

Liaison role of the nurse

Efficient communication with other district nurses is essential, including full and useful notes. 'GNC' given is totally inadequate and is unfor-tunately seen too frequently. Night nurses staying with the patient for the last few nights can often make the difference between death at home and a moribund patient being transported to hospital. This service may be provided by an agency nurse funded partly by the local authority and partly by the Marie Curie Foundation. Some districts will have direct access to Marie Curie nurses, others have a 24-hour nursing service and provide their own night sitters. This can have disadvantages. If the dis-trict is unduly busy the night sitter may only spend a very few hours with the patient or there may be more patients requiring a night nurse than the number available. This leads to uncertainty for the family and increases anxiety. Again communication between day and night nurses needs to be carefully co-ordinated.

Recreational therapy is vital in the home as much as in hospital. Patients feel frustrated by their weakness and a burden to their family. It is important to encourage a useful activity so that they feel they are con-tributing to society. A recreational therapist can usually decide what is appropriate for each patient. 'Live until you die' is a useful expression in these circumstances.

Many patients benefit from visits by the clergy and this should be arranged if required. It is important not to pressurize the patient with religion which may not be welcome. Social workers are an integral part of the team (see Chapter 13). Briefly, they are invaluable for making sense of complicated financial tangles in which some families find themselves. They can produce relatively rapid miracles by bringing forward a telephone installation or discovering a grant of money for a family in debt.

Their principal function before and after the death is to unravel some of the psycho-social problems; to anticipate and plan to prevent further distress, for example to single-parent families. The social worker's shoulder is often also invaluable for other professionals caring for the patient! The fresh view or insight a social worker can bring to a situation is often very different from that of a nurse or doctor.

The intrepid home help service can also make the difference between a patient coping at home or not. If the patient lives alone the home help may be the main carer.

Physiotherapists can be very helpful for gentle rehabilitation, exercises and massage. Gentle chest physiotherapy and postural drainage may be the treatment of choice for a dying patient with a chest infection. The ingenuity of the physiotherapist is often stretched to produce interesting-looking pieces of equipment out of foam rubber or polystyrene –whatever necessary to improve patient comfort.

An occupational therapist may be involved to make minor home adaptations such as improved stair bannisters or bath rails. Complicated, expensive and lengthy alterations are usually not appropriate for the dying.

The nurse must liaise with the general practitioner, who may have known the patient and family for many years. Sometimes, however, the doctor may believe there is nothing he can do and so feels awkward visiting the patient. The nurse may tactfully indicate that the patient would be pleased to see the doctor anyway – and this is indeed so. It may also be necessary for the nurse to apply persistent persuasion if the patient's pain and other symptoms are not adequately controlled. Any hospice would be happy to give telephone advice to a general practitioner, and may be available for domiciliary visiting.

If a patient needs a paracentesis, this can be done very simply by the doctor in the patient's home, using a peritoneal dialysis cannula plus receptacle for the drainage. This is done very successfully by some domiciliary hospice teams already. It saves an unnecessary trip to hospital or even admission for the procedure.

Local volunteer agencies may provide extra company to sit with the patient, thereby enabling the spouse to go shopping or to the dentist, or simply to have a break from the house.

Meals-on-wheels service may be needed occasionally for patients living alone. The special local laundry service, if available, is not often needed because by the time the patient becomes incontinent he usually has only a few days to live. If the patient is admitted to hospital or hospice it is always helpful to send an explanatory note, however brief, with the patient. It is important to provide enough information about the patient's condition to make the transition less traumatic. If a relative is able to accompany the patient this should be encouraged.

References

Simpson, M A (1979) The Facts of Death (chap. 2: 17), Prentice-Hall

Williamson, J (1979) The challenge, in D Doyle (Editor) Terminal Care, Churchill Livingstone

CHAPTER 10

CARE OF DYING PATIENTS IN HOSPITAL – SPECIAL ASPECTS
BARBARA SAUNDERS

Why should this type of care be any different from caring for a patient in a hospice? The answer is, of course, that it need not be different but there are important aspects in teaching and changing of attitudes that can make all the difference between a patient dying peacefully and one whose death is disturbed.

This chapter will describe, using St Thomas' Hospital Support Team as a model, how staff can be taught to care for dying patients amongst the everyday happenings of a busy ward; how nurses and doctors can come to terms with death and dying and go on to teach others; how relatives can be encouraged to take on the caring of the patient at home, so long as they are able. Finally, this chapter will comment on the needs of dying patients in specialist areas and the staff who care for them.

Teaching staff in a busy ward to care for dying patients

In December 1977, a team – consisting of a consultant and her registrar, both radiologists, working in their spare time, a full-time sister, a part-time social worker and the hospital chaplain – was formed to advise nurses and doctors at St Thomas' Hospital in London (Bates et al. 1981; Saunders 1980) how to control the symptoms of patients suffering from terminal malignant disease.

The hospice movement had been in operation locally for about 10 years and a considerable number of nurses, doctors and medical students had visited and been taught at St Christopher's Hospice. Despite this education, it was observed in the hospital and in the community that patients were still suffering pain and other distressing symptoms from their cancers.

Whilst nurses and doctors did care and agreed with the basic principles of keeping their patients symptom free and alert, they found it difficult to put them into practice without careful guidance. Many were apprehensive about the use of strong analgesia. They had seen evidence of the misuse of drugs amongst patients coming to casualty, and had read about it in the press.

These staff needed to be taught how symptoms could be controlled, as well as keeping their patients alert, with the added satisfaction of seeing most patients go home. They needed to understand addiction and whether it would affect these particular patients. The World Health Organization defines addiction as: 'A state, psychic and sometimes physical, resulting from the interaction between a living organism and a drug, characterized by behavioural and other responses that always include a compulsion to take the drug on a continuous periodic basis in order to experience its psychic effects, and sometimes to avoid the discomfort of absence.'

Dying patients require their pain to be controlled and do not require the drugs for their psychic effects. In fact, if pain is stopped by other means, then analgesia can be reduced and sometimes discontinued without ill effect. Nurses and doctors were interested in various drugs that could be used – how long their effect was maintained. They needed to understand that dosages needed to be titrated against the pain and to know the side-effects of these drugs. Such drugs need not be abandoned because once or twice the result was unpleasant or ineffective, but that some drugs were inappropriate.

As a Team, our mode of action is to visit patients, at the request of their consultant, on the day of referral. It is important to start by discussing the patient with the nurse in charge, and the ward doctor if available, and to read the patient's medical history. Armed with this information one Team doctor and the sister introduce themselves to the patient. With the patient's permission we sit down and encourage him to talk about his problems as he sees them, to recount his illness and his social background and to ask questions if he so desires. It is important that on this occasion the patient is given time so that a sense of trust begins to be built. At the end of the interview it is explained to the patient what we are going to suggest to his doctors and nurses, that we are only giving an opinion and not taking over his care and that we, or perhaps just the sister, will return each day.

The next stage is to write down the problems as the patient sees them in his casenotes and suggest solutions. Discussion with the ward staff is again important. Sometimes suggestions about the nursing care of the patient, tactfully given, are important. For instance, a lemon mouthwash may be more refreshing for somebody who can hardly swallow. Crushed ice-cubes to suck may be easier to manage than a drink. The dietitian's help may be sought when eating or drinking is difficult. The loan of an angle pillow, 'Spenco' mattress, heel or elbow pads, may make the patient more comfortable. The question of why temperatures are being taken and fluid balance charts maintained can also be discussed. The assistance of the diversional therapist or librarian could be sought, or an appointment made with the hairdresser. At the same time it is important for the nurse in charge to know that the Team sister, who might be seen as a threat to her authority, only wants to help the patient to be free of symptoms and to be given the best quality of life for the time he has left. She also wants the nurse to understand that caring for the terminally ill can be satisfying, but that it is stressful, and the Team sister is there to give any help or advice if it is needed.

When staff are frantically busy it is appropriate for the Team sister to offer practical help for a dying patient: perhaps by sitting and holding the dying patient's hand or by feeding another in a leisurely fashion; helping to make a bed; taking a prescription to pharmacy; collecting a book from the library; or just sitting and chatting. These small actions may help the patient, but they will also teach the nurses how care is put into practice.

The patient is revisited daily during his hospital stay. Following visits need not be so long, but if a patient trusts us and wants to ask questions, then the visit may be longer. Gradually we may learn what the patient knows about his illness and what else he wants to understand.

We need to interpret his gestures, pick up clues or cues, verbal or non-verbal, and be ready with honest answers in language he can understand, sometimes illustrated by a simple drawing. This information must be written in patients' notes and explained to the nurse in charge, often encouraging her to learn how to give further information if questions are asked.

By observing a patient whose symptoms are gradually being controlled, nurses and doctors begin to see how they can do this themselves, first with assistance and then alone.

One of the first results of the Team's work at St Thomas' was to alter the attitude of prescribing the old 'Brompton Cocktail'. A previous attitude might have been that the pain of the final stages of cancer simply meant prescribing 'Bromptons', implying that no more could be done for the patient. It was prescribed mostly with little imagination and usually had the same ingredients, diamorphine 10 mg, cocaine 5 mg, chlorpromazine 25 mg, alcohol, honey or syrup to 10 ml, irrespective of need. If this mixture did not control pain, injections were given, and if they did not keep the patient and nurses quiet, then increasing doses of sedation were added. This was given not because the doctors and nurses did not care, but because they had not been better informed.

We tried to teach nurses and doctors a better way to prescribe a simple diamorphine mixture in chloroform water, to add an anti-emetic if required, to give it regularly, 4-hourly, and to titrate the strength of the analgesia against the patient's pain. We also taught that there was no virtue in pain, as some might have thought; that our patients had chronic pain, not the type of acute or postoperative pain that staff, particularly on surgical wards, were familiar with.

We also needed to explain that the pain of bony secondaries was best controlled with the antiprostaglandin type drug, such as aspirin, indomethacin or phenylbutazone (Butazolidin), and that this could be given as well as diamorphine.

Pain in its various types needed to be explained: as well as physical pain, the patient perhaps had social or mental pain. Nurses are in a unique position to ferret out particular problems and to try to solve them, sometimes with the help of the chaplain or social worker.

At a later stage we began to introduce other analgesic drugs into our teaching, such as buprenorphine and slow-release morphine sulphate. These different drugs caused other teaching problems in that staff needed to have explained the different ways they worked; that a 4-hourly regime was not appropriate and that other regular analgesia could not be used with buprenorphine (as it is a partial opiate antagonist). It is important, however, in hospital to use new drugs and not to be complacent about just using the well-tried 'friend'. By using them we may find better ways of making our patients' lives more tolerable as well as relieving nurses of unnecessary tasks.

It is also important for nurses to know that drugs can be given by other routes apart from the mouth. Suppositories are extremely useful if a patient cannot swallow, or is vomiting. Analgesic drugs, such as oxycodone, morphine and diamorphine, and non-steroidal anti-inflammatory drugs, like aspirin, indomethacin and phenylbutazone (Butazolidin), come in suppository form; as do the anti-emetics, chlorpromazine and prochlorperazine. Another drug which has been produced in this form is diazepam, which seems, from our experience, to be more effective rectally than by injection. When regular analgesia can only be given by injection, the syringe driver is very helpful (Russell 1979 and see Note on p. 75). This delivers a steady subcutaneous infusion over 24 hours.

When a dying patient's symptoms are well controlled, nurses do not seem to be so concerned about nursing him in a separate room. Some patients prefer to stay in the ward. It is sometimes beneficial for other patients to observe a patient dying peacefully and to know that the nurses are watching him carefully and that relatives are encouraged to stay. It is equally good for other patients to be nursed in a single room, particularly when relatives want to stay all the time, and to be involved with the care. This is especially relevant when a patient has been nursed at home but has had to be readmitted for the last few days of his life. To encourage a family to continue to help at this stage can be very beneficial in their bereavement.

Apart from teaching in a practical way day by day, it is essential to have the opportunity for classroom teaching, because not all nurses work on wards where we are invited to advise.

Classroom teaching was originally given to trained staff so they could understand why the Team was involved with only some patients. They were taught how symptoms could be controlled and the importance of our Team advising rather than taking over, in order to teach other nurses and doctors to care in the future and to avoid confusion amongst patients.

The next group to be taught were nurses in introductory block. It is important for them to discuss the fact that patients do die – everybody does one day; that dying is not a failure, and although it is sometimes sad, it does not need to be depressing, so long as patients die peacefully, with symptoms well controlled. It is helpful for them to suggest the nursing problems that may be encountered in the care of this group of patients and how they will be able to alleviate them. Often this is the first time these young people have discussed death.

At a later stage nurses are taught about symptoms and how they can be controlled and we discuss whether in fact this is happening in the hospital. It would be useful if medical students could join nurses during this lecture; they are going to work together in the future and to discuss such an important topic together could be very advantageous.

It is important that all newly appointed nurses and doctors learn that a Team exists in the hospital, how we can be contacted and our mode of action.

Teaching also takes place in seminars on the wards. On these occasions particular patients can be discussed; we talk about problems and whether they were overcome or not. It is an opportunity for nurses to voice their feelings, anger, frustration, sadness or satisfaction. We can also discuss other patients who have gone home and who are enjoying a relatively good quality of life, and others who have died peacefully with their families at home.

Although not every acute general hospital will have introduced a support team to assist staff in the manner described, many ward sisters have found that the practice of allocating nurses to care for individual patients as far as possible, rather than task allocation, does help to ensure positive attitudes towards the needs of the dying patient and the sorting out of priorities, even in a ward with many different competing pressures on the staff. Some nurses find that when the principles of the Nursing Process are being applied in their ward it is also a help towards providing emotional as well as physical care to a dying patient and the family.

But whichever process is adopted it remains of paramount importance to ensure that the patient's symptoms are controlled. The sister needs to have knowledge of how this can be achieved, so she is able to advise the doctor if the need arises.

Coming to terms with death and dying and teaching others

When symptoms are controlled nurses feel much more at ease with their patients. When the patient has a symptom that the nurse is powerless to control, the temptation is to ignore the patient, or to spend little time with him. Nurses and doctors do not feel unhappy at using strong analgesia if they see patients alert and mobile, with their pain controlled, able to return home and sometimes resume employment.

Staff do not fear dying if they see patients die peacefully, knowing that if an unpleasant symptom does arise there is a Team within the hospital whose advice can always be sought.

Being honest with patients about the nature of their illnesses and passing this information on to other members of staff, can only make for a more relaxed atmosphere in which to work.

If staff are content that patients are really comfortable, they are able to discuss with relatives in a more straightforward way, what is going on and why. They are also able to encourage them to continue this caring at home, with help from community staff.

Nurses and doctors who have learnt good terminal care can teach their juniors by example in the wards. They can also take this knowledge to other wards, where perhaps these skills are not so widely practised. Finally when they leave the hospital, they can take this expertise to other hospitals, knowing that if they look after patients with symptoms that are not easily controlled, they can always refer back to the Team for further advice.

Some nurses and doctors will still find it difficult to come to terms with dying, and perhaps this is because they cannot contemplate their own deaths.

Teaching relatives how to continue with care at home

Relatives will usually only consider taking a patient home to die if most symptoms are controlled. They are often very apprehensive and need to be approached gently. Very few families these days have observed a person dying, except dramatically or violently on television. They therefore have no reason to think dying will be any different in reality.

The nurse in charge needs to explain about the advantages of going home, if that is what the patient wants; how drugs are given and how often – a clearly written instruction card is a help. She needs to enquire whether help will be required at home, whether the patient will have to use stairs. She may suggest bringing his bed into the living room. She should know the height of the bed at home – practising getting in and out of one of similar height in hospital will ensure that it can be done safely. She should ask where the toilet is: the loan of a commode may be helpful; whether the patient is going to require a community nurse to assist in his care, or, if the family want to do the nursing themselves, whether they are capable of it; whether a home help or meals-on-wheels would be needed and if financial assistance can be obtained. Questions such as these can be answered with the help of a social worker.

When a patient known to the St Thomas' Support Team is going home, one of the doctors contacts the patient's general practitioner, to see whether he is agreeable to one of the community nurses working in our Team continuing to support the patient and family at home. (Our nurses are attached to the District Service, but work similarly to the hospital sister, in an advisory capacity with the district nurses.) If permission is given, we are able to give the patient and relative telephone numbers and explain that if advice is needed, somebody is always on call. This is a great reassurance to relatives, who perhaps have had difficulty in the past in obtaining help. Many are reluctant to ask advice of a doctor, fearing the question may be regarded as stupid, but feel more able to ask a nurse.

It is also important to let the family know that should they be unable to continue the care, the patient will be able to be readmitted. It may be necessary to discuss the possibility of admission to a hospice at some stage.

At times it is useful to send a patient home for a trial day, or week-end, to find snags which can then be solved before a final discharge. When a patient is going home to be alone, an occupational therapy assessment and home visit before discharge are very useful.

Nurses and relatives need to make careful plans before a terminally ill patient is discharged home. Experience has shown that a hastily discharged ill patient soon returns to hospital.

Caring for the old person who is dying in hospital

For these patients we need to consider a longer time-span, generally speaking, and to discuss quality of life and how that can be maintained (British Geriatric Society and Royal College of Nursing 1975).

If the geriatric patient is dying from malignant disease then the same principles should be followed as already mentioned. Of the patients we care for at St Thomas' 60% are over 65 years of age.

Many geriatric patients die from arteriosclerotic disease, perhaps the terminal stage being a sudden coronary thrombosis. Usually it is inappropriate to resuscitate such patients but rather to ensure that they are pain free, not left alone and that relatives are fully informed of the situation. Others have a series of cerebrovascular accidents, perhaps none very severe but each leaving him in a weaker state. How important it is that the patient's dignity is maintained, that he is dressed in his own clothes, that attention is given to hair, teeth and nails, that he is encouraged to be as independent as possible. Pneumonia may be his final illness, which should not be treated with antibiotics, but by Tender Loving Care. He should be turned frequently, his mouth kept clean, and sips of iced water given. He may become hot and sweaty, when cotton nightclothes will be cooler; his own rather than the hospital variety will look more pleasant. The use of a fan will make him more comfortable. If he becomes 'bubbly' then an injection of hyoscine 0.2–0.4 mg given 6-hourly will dry the secretions and quieten him. If he is anxious, diazepam or chlorpromazine by suppository 8-hourly will relieve this symptom.

When geriatric patients are dying in hospital, or old people's homes, it is important to explain to their friends what is happening. They may have known him for a long while and may want to sit with him and say goodbye. They will be realizing that their own deaths may not be far away and observing a friend die peacefully, with good care, can serve to make them less afraid.

Many old people have been brought up with far more respect for, and interest in, Christianity than the present generation and it is important that they are offered a visit by the minister or priest.

Some of the nurses will have become very fond of their patients, whom they may have looked after for a long while. These nurses should be given opportunities to talk about their sadness. They and some of the other patients may wish to attend the funeral. This should be encouraged as a useful outlet for grief. Perhaps flowers from the funeral will be sent to the home or ward, so that they can be enjoyed by the remaining patients and staff.

Caring for the dying patient in intensive care units

Nurses caring for these patients are often under additional strain because:

1 The patients are often young.

2 The nurses and doctors have been working under extreme pressure to cure the patient and death will feel like utter failure.

3 The death is sometimes very soon after admission and the family will be extremely shocked and distressed.

4 The medical team will be caring for other patients who are similarly acutely ill, possibly in the same area.

How does the nurse care in this very clinical atmosphere, electric with anticipation? She has to remember that she is looking after a human being, albeit attached to many pieces of equipment, who can usually hear what she says, and the way that she says it, although he may not be able to answer. He can probably feel her caring hands, although he may not be able to move. A patient, who may be in pain or have other needs and be unable to shout, requires his nurse's senses to anticipate his needs and alleviate them. All this is stressful and requires a nurse to have special qualities.

The nursing team needs to be headed by a person with great sensitivity to the feelings of her staff. She needs to comfort, explain, encourage and show concern for her staff and the relatives as much as care for her patients.

It is important for doctors and nurses working in intensive care to have opportunities to discuss patients in team meetings, with other specialists to help them, such as a psychologist, chaplain and social worker.

Caring for the terminally ill patient with renal disease

Staff must cope with the problem of deciding not to treat some renal patients or abandoning dialysis treatment. Another problem is the disappointment of patient, relatives and staff following kidney transplant rejection. The patient will probably have been known in the renal department for many years; he and his family may have become friends of the staff.

The same principles apply in end-stage renal failure as in terminal cancer. The symptoms must be controlled in the best way possible and the patient and his family given help and support in a kind and understanding fashion.

The patient will be lethargic and drowsy, so the nurse, or perhaps a relative, will need to give help with his general care, allowing him to keep as much independence as he is able to cope with.

If his appetite is poor, it is important that his meals should be small and attractively presented. Keeping to a rigid diet is inappropriate; rather he should be allowed to eat and drink what he fancies.

He will often be nauseated, which may be relieved by cyclizine 50 mg given twice daily. If he also has hiccups, then chlorpromazine will relieve this symptom as well as the nausea. It can conveniently be given by suppository, if this route is acceptable to the patient.

If the patient has pain then this should be relieved in the most appropriate way; there is no point at this stage in withholding potent analgesia, if it relieves symptoms.

His skin may be dry and itching: arachis oil will relieve dryness; crotamiton (Eurax) cream may relieve the itching.

Mouth care is extremely important, because his mouth will be very dry and his gums may bleed. He may also develop Monilia, which will be relieved by nystatin suspension or miconazole (Daktarin) gel.

Another problem which may be very distressing to the patient and his family is realizing there is no drainage from a catheter, in which case removal should be considered.

The patient may also have fits, or muscle-twitching, which can be controlled by diazepam 5–10 mg given 8-hourly.

Relatives, the patient and staff need to be kept fully informed as to why medicines are given and how they will help, and if they do not relieve a symptom, they should be stopped.

Staff will sometimes be very distressed after such a patient dies and should be given the opportunity to talk about their sadness as well as successes, and to discuss the preventive side of the illness.

Conclusion

In conclusion, dying patients can be cared for in hospital just as well as in a hospice, so long as nurses pay attention to the details of basic care in a sensitive way and doctors prescribe appropriately. These combined efforts will lead to better care and job fulfilment.

References

Bates, T et al. (1981), Lancet I: 1201–1203

British Geriatric Society and Royal College of Nursing (1975) Improving Geriatric Care in Hospital

Russell, P S B (1979) Syringe driver, BMS, 9 June: 1561 (correspondence)

Saunders, B (1980) Terminal care support team, Nursing, July: 657

CHAPTER 11

CARE IN A HOSPICE – SPECIAL ASPECTS
SISTER ANTHONIA O'CONNOR and
SISTER PAULA GLEESON

A current definition of hospice is a community of people devoting their time exclusively to the care of dying patients, and sometimes the frail elderly and chronic sick or disabled as well. The term is not synonymous with a special building; hospice type of care may be given in a patient's home or in a ward set apart for the purpose in a general hospital.

Hospice care of dying patients, for whom the goal of cure is now inappropriate, aims to offer a complete service in which the emphasis is on freeing the person from distressing symptoms and ensuring that those caring for him have the time, skills and compassion to effectively support the patient until his death, and the family throughout this time and in their bereavement.

It has been pointed out that the dying patient and his family can also be given excellent care in an acute hospital ward. This, of course, is true but because of many conflicting needs staff can find it difficult to achieve what they wish to provide. Time may be lacking, personnel in short supply and the physical environment deficient in various ways. Doctors and nurses working in the community may also be frustrated in their desire to give a high-quality service to dying patients for similar reasons.

Those who have worked in hospices for a number of years have been able to build up a fund of knowledge and understanding, backed up by research, precisely because the resources are available for them to devote all their time to this field of care. Their expertise is being increasingly shared with other professional health workers; thus hospices can act as resource centres for improving the care of dying patients over a wider sphere.

Special features of hospice provision for residential care

The wards should be bright and cheerful in colour and design; the ideal basic size seems to be a 4-bedded unit, with some single rooms for those whose condition makes this more suitable, with their agreement. Large windows where patients can see people and traffic moving, if they are used to an urban environment, give a feeling of unity with the living world. Country dwellers, on the other hand, will appreciate being surrounded by beautiful natural scenery.

Unrestricted visiting is encouraged, since the patient and his family need frequent contact with each other. Relatives and friends should feel welcomed, and their physical and emotional comfort considered.

Reception and admission

When the patient, sometimes accompanied by relatives, arrives at a hospice, it is the custom for the trained nurse in charge to greet the patient at the entrance and escort him to his own ward where she will be responsible for his care. In this way, the patient is treated as a true guest with courtesy and a warm welcome. It is common for the nurse to be with the relatives while the doctor is taking a history from the patient, and examining him. This can be an opportunity for anxious and sad relatives to unburden themselves to a sympathetic listener. If they have been looking after the patient at home, there may be an expression of guilt at not being able to continue, and a feeling of failure. They are likely to be very tired, and apprehensive as to how the patient will come to terms with his new environment. The nurse should ensure privacy whilst interviewing the relatives, and provide comfortable chairs for them. The atmosphere should be unhurried to enable the nurse to obtain the necessary details about the patient (these can be added to later). Some type of nursing history sheet should be used, which will also be of value to doctor, social worker and other professional members of the caring team, for instance the physiotherapist. A very important need is to have the family's views on the degree of insight that the patient has into his condition. This may be stated spontaneously, and accompanied by a stipulation as to what the family considers the patient should be told, or not told.

The doctor will also wish to meet the relatives to ensure that they have an accurate understanding of the situation, and there may be a pressing reason why the social worker should be involved at an early stage. Unless the patient is near to death on admission, which can be the case, the relatives will want to see the patient settled before they go home, and should be offered a cup of tea, sitting with the patient. The usual precaution of obtaining a telephone number should be taken, and assurance given that the relatives are welcome to telephone or call whenever they wish.

A significant feature of hospice care, and one that has already been mentioned, is that time is made available to spend with patients not only when some physical procedure needs to be carried out, but at other times, simply providing companionship and a willingness to listen. This means that an adequate ratio of staff to patients is essential. Follow-up care of bereaved families is an important service, developed mainly by social workers, often with a team of trained volunteers. However, nurses have a part to play here because they will often have built up a close relationship with the family of a dying patient and may attend the funeral. They can help with the follow-up care by inviting the family to feel welcome to call into the ward from time to time to maintain contact.

Finally, the fact that hospices are relatively small in comparison with general hospitals helps to foster a sense of close community among staff which will be sensed by patients and relatives. Rigid hierarchical barriers are out of place, and consultation and sharing of problems is beneficial to patients and staff.

It is essential for a hospice to be situated near a general hospital where facilities such as an X-ray department (and radiotherapy), clinical laboratories and dentistry are available. The need for such technical assistance will not occur frequently, but can bring considerable relief on occasion to individual patients. For instance, a single dose of radiation therapy can bring dramatic reduction of pain for a patient with malignancy of bone.

The pace of life in a hospice is much more relaxed than in the large general hospital. Staff will try to go at the patient's pace rather than follow their own inclination, and to aim at an informal and homely style of ward management. There should be opportunities for patients to go home for a day or a week-end if they wish, provided the family can cope and no extra strain or burden will be put upon them. This requires consultation between doctor, nurse and social worker before finalizing the matter with the patient and family.

The homely quality of a hospice is enhanced by the absence of a multiplicity of charts hanging on beds, by little or no evidence of intravenous infusions, and by the freedom from the inevitable bustle and noise of trolleys taking patients to and from operating theatre or other departments. All this activity is necessary and justifiable in institutions devoted to cure as well as care, but it is an inappropriate intrusion into the peaceful surroundings of dying patients in a hospice.

Because of the considerable interest being shown at present in hospice work, both by professionals and the lay public, there are many requests to be 'shown round'. This commendable interest must be channelled in a suitable way, as too many groups or individual visitors walking through the wards can be an excessive invasion of the privacy due to dying patients and their families, and a strain for staff. It is usually preferable to arrange talks illustrated with slides or a film showing the work of the hospice, and keep tours to a minimum. This is usually accepted with understanding, particularly when it is explained that it is not customary to isolate the patient and family behind screens during the last hours of life.

The inpatient care of a hospice is usually combined with a home care service. The latter is often known as a Macmillan Service, being supported by the National Society for Cancer Relief (NSCR). This requires close co-operation and efficient communication between all staff so that if and when a patient is admitted for inpatient care, the home care team are able to keep in touch with how the situation progresses until the patient returns home. The main reason for admission is to give the caring family a temporary respite from their responsibilities; or there may be other social reasons. Sometimes, naturally, the patient deteriorates and dies in the hospice.

The qualities which go into the making of a hospice are not exactly definable. Samuel C. Klagsbrun states that although a hospice need not be a religious organization, it would seem essential that there is a spiritual dimension to its structure – to the rational human being, suffering and death ultimately have to make sense in order for the person to remain human (1981).

History of the hospice movement

The word 'hospice' has its origin in the Roman word 'hospes' – meaning both a host and a guest. From this tradition of hospitality, both hospitals for treatment of the sick, and hospices for giving temporary help and accommodation to travellers and care to the dying developed. Hospitals can be traced back to the ancient world, but the dominant influence in the growth of hospices was Christianity (although the two concepts were interchangeable for several centuries).

Most of the credit for early hospices must be attributed to the Knights Hospitallers of the Order of St John of Jerusalem. These were founded in Malta in 1065, primarily for the task of caring for the sick and dying on pilgrimage to and from the Holy Land.

At the peak of their flowering, records show an attitude of great consideration and respect for the needs of the individual – what would be called today a holistic approach to care. The same was true of the mediaeval hospices operating throughout Europe; 750 were in existence in England alone.

Following the suppression of the monasteries and the dispersal of religious men and women, the sick, poor and dying were left without help and medicine and nursing remained at a low ebb for a considerable time, hospitals at that period being a place to be dreaded and avoided at all costs.

The modern hospice

It was not until the middle of the nineteenth century that the old idea of the hospice began to revive. The Sisters of Charity, founded by Vincent de Paul in 1600, had worked quietly for three centuries among the poorest and most despised members of French society, and during the nineteenth century influenced such pioneers as the Protestant pastor Fliedner (who founded Kaiserswerth), Florence Nightingale and Elizabeth Fry.

In 1840 an Irishwoman, Mary Aikenhead, opened in Dublin a place of shelter and care for the incurably ill and dying and called it by the old mediaeval name of 'hospice'. She founded a new order of nuns, the Irish Sisters of Charity, who in 1906 opened a similar house in London – St Joseph's Hospice, which has continued until the present day in caring for dying patients and those with chronic illnesses. Just before the opening of St Joseph's Hospice, two other hospices had opened in London – St

Luke's, started by the Methodist West London Mission (now closed), and the Hostel of God, started by Anglican Sisters. The latter closed for several years, but is now operating under lay administration and has been renamed Trinity Hospice.

While this development was proceeding in Europe, a parallel revival of the old hospice ideal was taking place in America, through the work of a Dominican order of nuns founded by Rose Hawthorne. Their first hospice opened in New York in 1899, and was followed by others. In the 1950s an important development was the establishment of the Marie Curie Foundation, which aimed to relieve the distress of patients dying with cancer, and the strain on their families. Homes were set up to provide hospice care. The highest point of the hospice movement in this century so far was reached through the work of Cicely Saunders. In revolutionizing the approach to control of pain and other distressing symptoms in dying patients and in re-emphasizing the right of the patient to a peaceful and dignified death, she has led the way and inspired others to introduce hospice care all over this country and in North America.

At St Joseph's Hospice, where she was appointed as the first full-time medical officer, and began her special work for dying patients, she was able to build on the tradition and practice of loving care carried out for more than half a century by this Christian community, whose original priority had been relieving the distress caused by wide-spread tuberculosis in East London. Many of the victims died at home or in the hospice, tended by the Sisters. In then founding St Christopher's Hospice in 1967, Cicely Saunders drew together the threads of care traced back over nearly 2000 years, and enriched the work with a new emphasis on scientific research and teaching.

Present and future trends

In the United Kingdom, there are now at least 100 hospice programmes in existence, and more in the planning stage. Much financial help and guidance continues to be given by the NSCR, with particular emphasis on home care support teams – the Macmillan Services. These are specialist teams working closely with the primary care teams. Most hospices are largely independent, but the NSCR has developed an approach of helping to build and equip a number of units in the grounds of NHS hospitals and then handing them over to the particular district health authority whose responsibility they have become. Hospice units tend to be relatively small in size, say between 12 and 25 beds, in comparison with the older hospices such as St Joseph's and St Christopher's.

With the much greater interest in the needs of dying people and their families, both by the health care profession and the general public, the whole subject has been opened up for research and debate. As the basic concepts of hospice care become more widely understood and applied in hospitals (where about 60% of people in the United Kingdom die), some believe that hospices should 'plan for [their] own obsolescence', linked with the provision of counselling, support and good symptom control for patients and relatives, upgrading of community terminal care, and a vigorous teaching programme for young doctors and nurses. This will result in a hospice having only a few beds, and not necessarily functioning in a special unit on its own, but as a centre associated with schools of medicine and nursing (Wilkes 1981). A detailed and well-documented analysis of the effectiveness of hospice care, including cost-benefit, is needed to justify separate hospice care (Torrens 1981). Finally, there is a challenge to be met in the application of hospice concepts to a broader section of care: since it has been widely accepted as having achieved much for dying patients, other groups such as chronic sick, mentally handicapped and the frail elderly deserve the same efforts to be made on their behalf.

Many countries throughout the world are giving much thought to the most appropriate way in which hospice-type care can be developed. In some countries, rather than build free-standing hospices, existing institutions are used in which an improved care service for dying people can be based. In others, particularly in the USA, there has been a great proliferation in home care programmes.

Some views expressed by patients and relatives in a particular hospice

The following are answers given by some patients when asked how they would describe a hospice:

'A home from home.'
'Not like a hospital – just like a beautiful big drawing-room. Full of loving people!'
'A place where I know I am wanted.'
'A place where people have time to listen.'

Although home is the ideal place in which to die, this is not always possible. A hospice can be a haven of peace for the patient and his family, particularly because of the lack of hurry and tension inevitable to some extent in an acute hospital ward.

Acceptance of death

Those of us whose privilege it often is to sit by the bedside of a dying patient know well that the moment of death need be neither frightening nor painful, but a peaceful end to the functioning of the body. This was brought home to me as I sat at the bedside of an only child – Ronnie – who was dying of cancer. His father and mother sat beside him praying silently. We seemed to be enveloped in an atmosphere of great peace. Ronnie was just 9 years old. Suddenly the silence was broken when his father said, 'Sister, we have had Ronnie for 9 wonderful years. We realize that he is only a loan from God; now we give him back. We shall be very lonely, but he is going to a better home and one day, please God, we shall join him.' This remarkable acceptance came after months of suffering – both parents rebelled at first and could not accept this cruel cross, but gradually they found peace.

Overcoming fear

For many people the thought of death and dying is fearful. The fear may relate to death itself – how it may come and what may be found after death. The practice in a hospice of not hiding the dying patient behind curtains during his or her last hours can have a calming and reassuring effect, as can be seen by the following incident.

Mrs X was a frail, worried little lady of 50 years. She knew that she was dying and was very frightened. A few days after admission to the hospice she said one morning, 'I am not afraid of dying now since I saw Dora slip away. [Dora was a patient in the opposite bed and they had become friends.] It was so beautiful – Dora had just had her hair done and she looked so pretty when suddenly she cried out that she felt queer and wanted Sister. Sister and doctor came, then the chaplain. They all knelt down and prayed. Sister held Dora's hand and she went so quietly and peacefully. I hope I go that way too.' Mrs X did 'go that way' a few days later.

This gentle passage from life to death can only be achieved if we have succeeded in a large measure in relieving any distressing symptoms of mind, body and spirit. Some patients will have lived their lives according to particular religious beliefs and will find comfort in the confidence of eternal life to which death is the awakening. The person with no belief in an after life may also die calmly and peacefully since to him when death comes all is over. The constant presence of a caring staff eager to give comfort and support to all without discrimination of race or creed must be the hallmark of a hospice.

Bereavement

Terminal care does not end with the death of the patient, whose sufferings are over – those of the family may be beginning. Professional support and help will be needed, and social workers in particular will visit the bereaved family or single relative. The custom that some of the hospice staff attend the funeral is much appreciated by relatives. A card sent by the hospice to the spouse or other close relative on the first anniversary of the death – simply saying 'We are remembering you' – is described by many as a great solace.

References

Cohen, K (1973) Hospice: Prescription for terminal care in (H), Aspen Publication

Klagsbrun, S C (1981) Hospice – a developing role, in C M Saunders et al. (Editors) Hospice: The living idea, Edward Arnold

Lamerton, R (1980) Care of the Dying, Pelican Books

Saunders, C M et al. (1981) Hospice – The living idea, Edward Arnold

Stoddard, S (1978 and 1979) The Hospice Movement, Vintage Books and Jonathan Cape

Torrens, P (1981) Achievement, failure and the future, in C M Saunders et al. (Editors) Hospice: The living idea, Edward Arnold

Wilkes, E (1981) Great Britain: the hospice in Britain, in C M Saunders et al. (Editors) Hospice: The living idea, Edward Arnold

CHAPTER 12

DYING CHILDREN AND THEIR FAMILIES
PEGGY COLLINGE and ELIZABETH D STEWART

The pronouncement that a child is terminally ill is one of the most difficult things for civilized man to accept. The older person is seen to have experienced life, to have known the joys as well as the trials of living; somehow it seems more acceptable, however unpleasant and sad. The child should be starting out in life, on the threshold of his existence. Few people can therefore ever come to terms with the death of a young person, although some find themselves in the position where they have no alternative.

Attitudes of parents

The parents for whom this is a reality require special understanding and management. A large proportion of children who die, do so as the result of accidents. This means that one minute the parents have an active, healthy offspring; the next he may be critically injured or even dead. These parents have no warning, no time in which to experience anticipatory grief. Many find the situation unbelievable; they may not absorb the details given by the medical staff, or they may even accuse them of exaggerating. It is not uncommon for them to become aggressive, accusing the hospital staff, as well as anyone involved in the actual accident, of being negligent and party to their child's death. Often these parents cannot believe their child is dying or dead until they see the little body lying lifeless in his bed. They are then devastated – sometimes so numb with grief that they show no outward signs of distress. Nurses find this extremely upsetting, particularly if they do not understand the reasons for the reaction. Other parents will become hysterical, whilst some will simply cry uncontrollably and inconsolably. The nurse needs to recognize that each individual parent has his or her own way of coping with this sudden disaster; she must not feel inadequate if she herself is shocked or unable to cope with such behaviour.

Few things can be worse for parents than to be told their child has a malignant disease or is terminally ill. Along with visions of pain and suffering are their own fears associated with the particular illness. (The media have a great deal to answer for in this respect.) The individual may be left emotionally distraught, unable to cope either with himself, his partner or his sick child. This in turn may be noticed by the child, who becomes frightened or depressed, not understanding his parents' reaction towards him. In order to provide adequate help and support for these parents, it is essential that the nursing staff get to know and understand them as individuals. Stanford B. Friedman stated in 1963: 'Each parent of a child with a fatal disease reacts to the tragedy in a unique manner, consistent with his personality structure, past experiences and the individualized meaning and specific circumstances associated with the threatened loss.' Until the nurse recognizes the implications for the individual parent, she will be unable to help him adjust to the situation and care for his child.

Certain reactions are to some extent predictable. In an era when it is unusual for a child to die, parents expect their offspring to live a full and active life. It is therefore extremely difficult for them to accept the diagnosis and prognosis, and they often experience an initial sense of shock and disbelief, sometimes lasting for several days. This provides a defence mechanism, allowing them time to begin to come to terms with the diagnosis. During this period, they may ask innumerable questions, not only of the hospital staff but of everyone available to answer them: friends, relatives, neighbours and even other parents on the ward. Some will obtain medical textbooks and read everything they can find pertaining to the disease. It is essential that the nursing staff make themselves available to talk to the parents at this time – despite the fact that the medical staff have explained everything, they will need to discuss the matter many times before accepting it. However, it is advisable for specific staff to support the parents throughout, as doubts may arise if different people describe the same course, treatment and prognosis in even slightly differing terms. The answers must at all times be consistent.

Following this 'questioning phase', there may be a period of absolute denial. Support by the hospital staff may be rejected, but must be readily available. The parents sometimes feel the diagnosis is incorrect, asking for a second opinion and further investigations. Once their initial denial gives way to acceptance, they frequently feel anger and guilt, directed towards the child, themselves and the medical/nursing staff involved. Their feelings towards their dying child are rarely manifest but nevertheless cause them even greater guilt reactions. In time, such feelings subside, and parents then invariably search for some meaning within the situation.

Throughout this difficult period in a family's life, the nursing staff can provide invaluable support. There are no answers as to how to deal with individual parents. Simply being with them and showing genuine concern will bring some solace.

Other relatives and friends

Even today, with fewer extended families, the majority of children have grandparents or other relatives. They must not be forgotten; their fears and grief may easily be as extensive as the child's parents'. Not only are they experiencing the tremendous sadness of knowing they will lose a beloved young relative, but they see his parents grieving also. Where possible, arrangements should be made for the entire family to be together with the child whenever they so wish. Facilities for resident parents and close relatives are therefore required; if these are not available, the family must be made to feel free to visit at any time, providing the child can cope with them. A granny or other loved one will provide comfort and security for the little one in mum and dad's absence, thus allowing them periods 'off duty'.

The opportunity to leave the child is particularly important if there are siblings at home. These youngsters will not fully comprehend what is happening to their family circle. The terminally ill brother or sister has probably been receiving more attention than usual, with one or both parents devoting themselves to his care and possibly even leaving the home to live in the hospital with him. The children may be old enough to realize that their sibling is ill, perhaps distressed and in pain. Hence, it is important that the parents explain the situation in terms the child can understand; even a small child will settle more readily if he has some idea of what is happening. He will need constant reassurance that his parents still love him, not loving his sibling in hospital any more than him. Eventually, the child will also have to come to terms with his brother or sister's death; he may not fully understand what dying means, but will realize that the child has not returned home. This may frighten him, whilst at the same time he will be aware of the sadness and distress of his parents and family. Frequently, the parents are too involved with the dying child to recognize these problems; the nursing staff have a duty to the family as a whole, to point out the potential difficulties and attempt to alleviate them whenever feasible. The parents need help to help their children.

School friends also require consideration. Although they will not be told the entire story during the child's illness, they need to realize he is ill and requiring special treatment to make him well. This is particularly important if the child is receiving steroids, leading to the characteristic change in appearance, or therapy causing alopecia. Otherwise the young patient may experience further suffering at the hands of his class mates. Once the child dies, these children must have the situation explained. It is not uncommon for others to fear they might have caught the fatal disease, or experience what they consider to be similar symptoms. With careful explanations, much anxiety can be avoided.

Psychological needs of the child

Many people find it difficult to know how to deal with the terminally ill child emotionally and psychologically. It is generally accepted that the child needs to know something about his illness, although the extent will depend on his age and understanding. To maintain his trust and confidence in the nursing and medical staff, it is important that knowledge is not withheld from the child but rather modified to suit his needs. It is very unusual for a child to ask 'Am I dying?', but, if he should do so, it must be remembered that in a child's understanding the word 'dying' can have various meanings. Children of varying ages have different experiences, ideas and fantasies; they may not therefore mean 'dying' as we understand it. Hence, if a child should ask, a way of handling the uneasy situation is to ask him what he means and what made him ask the question, why he should think he is dying, what it was that gave him the idea. The child should always be allowed time to think and talk openly; never rushed into answering, however uncomfortable the nurse herself may feel.

Usually this approach is enough; the child answers his own question and accepts his own answer. There are occasions, however, when the child appears to know and come to terms with his impending death without ever being told. Belinda aged 6 years had leukaemia. As a special treat she was taken for a day in the country and showed interest in the old village church. On entering, she noticed the children's corner and headed in its direction. There she sat on a small chair, looking up at a picture of Jesus surrounded by tiny angels. 'Where does Jesus get his little angels from? Are they children who have died?' she asked. This idea was confirmed by her adult escort, who pointed out that in reality very few children actually die. 'That's all right then,' said Belinda, 'I am going to be one of Jesus' angels soon, did you know that I am going to die soon?' Belinda died 6 weeks later, maintaining throughout this time that soon she too would be one of Jesus' angels.

The dying child will soon realize that he is taking longer to get well than other children. It is therefore helpful to introduce the idea that his particular illness is not one that can be treated and cured straight away but one which will take a long time, with various ups and downs to go through before he recovers. Long-term planning for the years to come, with talk of things which will happen when he is fit and strong again, also leads him to look to the future and tolerate his 'bad days' more easily. During the course of his treatment, the child will undergo a number of unpleasant or painful procedures. From the beginning it is essential that everything is explained to him; pain must never be denied. If the child asks whether a particular procedure hurts, he should be told it hurts a little bit, but the nurse will do it as quickly as possible and get it over with. This positive approach promotes his trust in the staff; the child knows he is being told the truth. Likewise, he must never be ridiculed for crying; he should always be praised for being brave, even if a few tears are shed. There is no place in paediatrics for the British stiff upper lip!

Recreation and activity

A child's normal activity is to play. Not only does he derive pleasure from it but it keeps his brain and hands active, providing an ideal diversion from the world around him. The terminally ill child needs to play as much as his healthy peers. Whilst the dying adult may simply lie in bed, not wanting to be occupied, the child should be encouraged to remain active for as long as possible. Obviously play activities will need to be modified according to the individual's condition, but the fact that the little one is in bed and sleeping much of the time does not mean that he should be left to lie quietly inactive during his periods of wakefulness. He may enjoy playing a game with a sibling or relative for short periods, or perhaps just looking at and talking about a favourite toy. Many children enjoy colouring pictures or drawing. Even if unable to do so himself, fun can be gained from watching an adult draw a picture of the child's choice, no matter how badly! Stories, the television, a record player, or simply being surrounded by other children and watching them play though unable to participate, will help to maintain the child's interest in life.

It must be remembered, however, that the child may wish to talk about his illness, feelings or fears. Play activities should therefore allow time and opportunity for such discussions, with the adult alert to cues which may be used to lead into it.

Even though the child is dying, normal discipline must not be totally abandoned. If the parents and staff give in to the youngster's every whim, it will not only lead to problems of management, but will make him feel insecure. If he has always been used to a particular code of conduct being demanded, he may wonder why this no longer applies. 'Am I dying perhaps?' Everyone must be aware of the things which are important to him, but should remain consistent in their attitudes and manner. Children are very astute and conscious of atmosphere; normality must therefore reign as far as possible. The parents and family will find this a daunting task, wishing to make amends to him for his short life. However, they must be assured that they are being kinder to him by behaving as normally as is humanly possible; not an easy fact for them to accept.

Pain relief and prevention

The paediatric nurse plays an important part in the pain relief of her patient. It must be remembered that the child may be too young to localize his pain, or perhaps unable to communicate the discomfort he is suffering. Tracy, a terminally ill 4 year old, complained of 'bad diarrhoea', although she suffered no such disorder. Eventually, after some hours, she was asked to describe what she meant. 'It's very bad,' she replied. 'It's in this ear and it hurts such a lot.'

Often the only way the little one has of expressing pain or discomfort is by crying; however, he may refuse to eat and drink, or appear 'difficult', withdrawn or unco-operative, refusing to conform to anything that is asked of him. His parents will find all of this distressing, maybe not realizing the reasons behind it. Careful explanations and support are required to alleviate their mental pain, as well as the measures necessary to help their child's physical pain. It is thus obvious that both parents and staff need to recognize the cues given by the individual child. Once this happens, the prevention and management become much easier. With children even more than adults, 'prevention of pain is better than cure'. An adult will understand the reasons for his pain; a little one will not. All he feels is lost and rejected by all around him. They are there but still allow him to experience such discomfort. This sometimes leads to the child rejecting those closest to him, blaming them for not helping in this time of need. Clearly, this adds to their distress. They feel helpless enough without additional anxieties.

The actual methods of providing pain relief for the youngster are in many ways the same as for the adult. The use of drugs and nursing management are fully covered in Chapter 6 and require only minor modifications. However, injections should be avoided wherever possible; the administration of intravenous analgesia via a cannula or infusion may be preferable to regular intramuscular injections. Oral preparations need to be flavoured adequately; many of them taste bitter and are therefore yet another unpleasant factor of life for the child. It is not uncommon for children to tolerate extreme pain rather than accept analgesia by injection or as a foul-tasting liquid.

We so often feel that we should find a position of comfort for a child in pain, but he will usually find out for himself what position gives most relief. The comfort of his mother's arms, where he can relax in security, will probably be his favourite place. When resting in bed, many children seem to need few covers, and often a sheet or light blanket loosely laid is best accepted. If he needs more warmth but cannot tolerate weight on his feet, a large soft toy pushed into position to take the weight of the blankets is often more acceptable than a conventional bed cradle. If he has difficulty breathing and prefers to be propped up, a very large teddy bear is comforting and supportive, and most stuffed toys are easily washed. A 'sag-bag' may also be useful in enabling him to participate in games on the floor while at the same time supporting him in his most comfortable position. Some children with breathing difficulty are more comfortable leaning forward over a firm support. They may find large washable floor cushions give just the support they need, 'sag-bags' filled with polystyrene beads are ideal for relieving pressure on aching limbs and sore skin.

The management and prevention of pain for the dying child are of paramount importance. Whether it is by the administration of regular analgesia (given before the previous dose wears off, not 'p.r.n.') or by specific nursing care, the objective remains the same: to alleviate the child's physical pain and reduce his loved ones' emotional pain.

Nutritional management

Nutritional management of the dying child requires careful consideration. There are numerous reasons why he may not be interested in eating and drinking or may even refuse food altogether. Some are associated with actual loss of appetite, but other factors must always be borne in mind.

Feeding the terminally ill child can present a problem especially for his mother, who feels that he has few reserves to fall back on. Obviously, he will be encouraged to keep to his normal routine for as long as possible and his eating pattern will be included in this routine. However, the time will come when he will be disinclined to eat a set meal at a pre-planned time. His mother may find that he is often asleep when meals are prepared, but that if he is allowed to eat what he fancies when he chooses, he may be able to maintain a reasonable level of nutrition. If the child is in hospital, it will be helpful if the mother can be offered facilities for cooking snacks. This will enable her to make a positive contribution to her child's care, and what child does not prefer his mother's cooking to institutional catering?

There are a number of commercial products available, both pleasing to taste and nutritious. Build Up and Complan are good examples. Unfortunately, their protein content may be too high for the toddler under two years if they are used in addition to other protein foods, and it is recommended that not more than two sachets per day are given to older children for the same reason. A very palatable, high-calorie milk, suitable for all children over one year, can be made by mixing one brickette of ice cream with two tablespoons of sugar and adding milk to make one pint. This can be used on cereals, or flavoured with syrups and milk shake powders as desired. Caloreen powder, which is tasteless, may be added to soups, yoghurt and savouries, or a high-calorie drink may be made by adding 7 level tablespoons of Caloreen to one pint of water and flavouring it with fruit juice as desired. This could even be frozen to make 'ice lollies'. Caloreen may be available on prescription. A dried skim milk powder such as Marvel added to soups is another way of increasing the child's protein intake, and double cream may be added to milk puddings and soups to increase calorie intake.

The mother of the child whose medical condition requires a special diet will obviously receive professional advice about meeting his particular needs. The doctor caring for the young patient can easily arrange an interview with the local dietitian.

Parental and family support

From the moment parents are told their child's diagnosis and/or prognosis, they may require support in excess of that which the ward team can provide. So many everyday living problems arise, far removed from the young patient himself. Whilst the family may have coped with home difficulties before, the news of their child's illness will pose additional stress. Even in the family unit without prior problems, a child's terminal illness will itself present untold misery within the home. The social worker therefore has an important role to play.

Most paediatric units have their own social worker, with special understanding of children and parents. The ways in which she may help include supporting the parents around the time they are given the diagnosis, then assessing their ability to cope with the long-term implications. She will have information available regarding the resources they may call upon, for example financial allowances, house adaptations and provision of nursing equipment for the home. The social worker can also assist the family with their hospital visiting, both whilst the child is an inpatient and once he attends the outpatients clinic. This can include helping to arrange the temporary care of siblings or advising on how to obtain money for fares, if hospital transport is not indicated. Another important role is to act as family confidante, supporting them emotionally through the traumatic period up to and including the child's death.

At times of heartbreak and distress, many people return to their religion. The nurse involved with terminally ill children of whatever faith must always offer this facility, regardless of her own beliefs and feelings. Sometimes the parents will reject the idea of any form of religious support, feeling that no God could allow their beloved child to die. However, many will find great solace in talking to the minister of their religion. It is always wise to ask the parents their feelings quietly and unobtrusively; the mere act of mentioning it may be all that is required to turn them to the invaluable support a chaplain can provide. Not only Christian children die, therefore it is essential to be sensitive to the beliefs and customs of all other faiths; information regarding their specific religious observances is readily available. It must be remembered that little things matter more to people and cause more distress than we ever realize.

Care of bereaved parents

As death approaches, the parents may again be struck with disbelief or anger and guilt. Their reactions are as unpredictable as the winds, but the nurse who has grown to know and understand them may recognize the way in which they are blowing. They should never be left to feel alone; although it is desirable for them to have the child to themselves for periods, the nurse should never be far away. It is often easier for her to cope with her own sadness if she avoids entering the room where the distraught relatives and dying child abide, but her presence is essential. The parents must be made aware that even though nothing further can be done for their little one, the hospital staff will go on caring even after he has died. It is preferable for the nurse to be in the room with them when the moment of death comes; they may be bewildered and frightened, not believing that the time has finally arrived for them to say goodbye for ever.

Following death, the parents may wish to have their child dressed in his best clothes and have a favourite toy left with him. This must be respected, although it may be easier for the undertaker to dress the body later. Once they are ready to leave, every effort must be made to provide support for them when they return home. Both the general practitioner and the health visitor should be notified, also the local vicar or who ever else they desire. The father's or mother's employer may be able to help, particularly if the parent has been away from work to be with the dying child.

The bereaved parents may require help and support for many months. There are a number of self-help groups available to provide such support. Cruse and the Society of Compassionate Friends co-ordinate their activities, and they will readily advise regarding where to go or whom to contact.

A bereaved parent: 'One of the hardest things is the sense of loneliness and isolation. Friends and even family, suddenly weren't around. They were embarrassed and felt inadequate. They didn't want to talk about Tony or his illness and it's worse since he died . . . .'

Conclusion

In this chapter we have attempted to put forward a few practical points which both nurses and parents might find useful.

It is a fact that with our present resources many children die in hospital rather than at home, but as paediatric nurses we recognize that this is far from ideal. The future success of extended community care is highlighted in the following quotation from Mother Frances Dominica (1982), founder of the first children's hospice, Helen House, Oxford:

I believe that a busy hospital is not the best place for a child to die, and if, therefore, the better arrangement is for the child to die at home, among familiar things and a caring family, then the role of the hospice emerges clearly: to act as support for this process, which conforms to the mediaeval concept of 'the good death' – living fully until the end and then passing away in peace, amidst family and friends. I believe that for many families this is a difficult and emotionally draining experience needing a greater measure of understanding and expert support, and above all a greater amount of time, than the services are always able to provide.

I recently lived in with a family for the last week of their young daughter's life. She held court downstairs in the sitting room until two days before the end, surrounded by her family and friends. Then, after two days, she died peacefully in her sleep. I believe that is the humane and dignified way to end a life, and however devoted the staff in a busy hospital, I know from my own experience that such an end is difficult to achieve.

References

Burton, L (1971) Cancer children, New Society, June

Burton, L (1974) Care of the Child Facing Death,

Dominica, Mother Frances (1982) The soothing touch, World Medicine, Aug

Evans, B (1976) The dying child, World Medicine, March

Friedman, S B (1963) Behavioural observations of parents anticipating the death of a child, Paediatrics, Oct

Jolly, J (1981) The Other Side of Paediatrics,

MacFarlane, I and N (1980) Nursing the dying child at home, Nursing Times, June

APPENDIX: THE NEEDS OF PARENTS FOLLOWING STILLBIRTH OR ABORTION   Margaret Linton

Stillbirth

Stillbirth is defined as a birth after the 28th week of pregnancy in which the baby does not breathe or show any other signs of life after being completely expelled from the mother.

The loss of the baby will be a profound shock and tragedy to the parents, and over the last 10 years there has been an increasing awareness of the grieving process involved in this special situation, and the importance of that process being allowed to take place. The grief reaction of the parents is thought to be the same as that following any bereavement – shock and denial, anger, guilt, depression and then acceptance – but there are difficulties for the parents of a stillborn baby because they are mourning a person who died before they physically met him. However, they may 'know' the baby in a deep instinctive sense. The mother will have felt him move and kick inside her, the father may have felt him move under his hand, and they will have been aware of him growing. It is not therefore helpful to tell parents that they can soon replace this particular baby by having another quickly. This devalues the baby, denies the reality of him, and belittles this shattering experience. If the parents are not helped to mourn their baby fully, it has been shown that relationship difficulties and problems with subsequent healthy children may develop.

Thus, parents should be helped through their grief and given the opportunity to express this. They should have the reasons for the baby's death fully explained to them and be given the chance to ask any questions they may have. They should be asked if they wish to see their baby and should have the opportunity to handle him. If the baby is not physically perfect it is usually possible to wrap him in an acceptable way so that his parents may see him. If the parents are denied this opportunity it may lead to exaggerated fears in their own minds about his physical appearance. If they do not wish to see the baby a photograph can be taken and kept in the records and the parents told of this in case they wish to see it at a later date. The parents may give consent to a postmortem and if this is held it is often an appropriate time, on receiving the report, for the doctor to go over again the circumstances leading to the loss and to explain the result, as the parents need time to absorb fully what has occurred. The parents are advised by the hospital staff about registration of the baby and subsequent funeral arrangements. These arrangements can be undertaken by the hospital or by the parents themselves and some parents do find it helpful to arrange a little funeral and give the baby a name, though this is not required by law.

Following delivery, mothers of stillborn babies have said they felt ashamed and embarrassed at being in a situation where other mothers and their babies are and this should be recognized and dealt with by the staff. The mother should be allowed to be where she feels most comfortable, whether it is with other mothers, or on her own, or at home as soon as she is fit to go. She should not be encouraged to rush home if that is not truly what she wants, as she may go home quickly in a state of shock to an anxious family who do not know how to cope with her and discourage her from grieving. Her general practitioner, community midwife and health visitor should be notified of the situation before she goes home, and she will be visited initially by the community midwife. Once home the parents will continue to need support and this can be provided by a professional person, such as a hospital social worker or a health visitor, or a support group such as the Stillbirth and Perinatal Death Association. The mother's 6-week post-natal check should not be carried out at a normal post-natal clinic with the bustle of mothers and babies, but either at a special counselling clinic or at a gynaecological clinic. Genetic counselling is usually given if appropriate, together with advice about future pregnancies. Couples are now usually advised to wait at least 6 months before embarking on another pregnancy, so that time to grieve fully is allowed. As with the loss of any loved person, the parents will never 'get over' the loss of their baby or forget him, but with help will usually be able to come to terms with their loss.

There is realization now that a stillbirth is a tragedy to the couple and their families, but there is still a need to recognize that it is also a tragedy to the mother's professional attendants, and they too can feel shock, anger and guilt. Unless medical and midwifery staff recognize and acknowledge *their* need to mourn this loss, they can never fully help the parents with their grief and be a support to them. They may, in fact, subtly reject the parents, becoming unwilling to talk to them, and wish to send the mother home quickly. Regular staff meetings with a skilled counsellor can be helpful, so that doctors and midwives can understand and acknowledge their own feelings and develop skills to help the parents more effectively in this situation.

Spontaneous abortion or miscarriage

Many women experience a painful sense of loss following a spontaneous abortion, and this form of bereavement should be treated with respect and the parents given the opportunity to express their hurt. Advice regarding other pregnancies and genetic counselling will be given, but it is important for professional staff to realize that for the couple concerned, this is the loss of their baby, and not just the passing of products of conception.

Termination of pregnancy

Another situation where grief may be very real is following a pregnancy that has been terminated. There is often either no opportunity to express this or the woman will hide it away, feeling that she cannot admit to her sense of loss. There may be guilt feelings immediately after the termination and a form of puerperal depression. Failure to cope with her feelings at this time may cause guilt and grief in a subsequent straightforward pregnancy, and therefore sensitive support and counselling at this time may be very helpful.

References

Copper, N E (1982) Stillbirth, Nursing, Feb: 1490

Health Education Council (1978) The Loss of Your Baby, Booklet published in conjunction with MIND and the National Stillbirth Study Group, obtainable from Health Education Council

Lewis, E (1976) The management of stillbirth: coping with an unreality, Lancet 2: 619–620

Pizer, H and Palinski, C (1980) Coping with Miscarriage: Why it happens and how to deal with its impact on you and your family, Jill Norman

CHAPTER 13

THE ROLE OF THE SOCIAL WORKER
JENNY PARDOE

Introduction

'Well, social work is largely a question of common sense isn't it?' said a nurse recently when I introduced myself as a social worker. This must be the comment that is most frequently heard, as we try to explain our role. There is undoubtedly a truth in the remark, but it is, surely, as relevant to nursing and many other forms of employment. Naturally, maturity, experience of life and a pragmatic approach help; where would they not?

Social workers become accustomed to being somewhat summarily dismissed in this way, especially by members of other caring professions. This may be because these other professions place greater emphasis on employing practical skills and knowledge which have a quantifiable result; my contention would be that there is nevertheless an inherent gap in such an approach by nature of the fact that our business is people, and ill people at that. People who are seriously or terminally ill are anxious, frightened, confused and overwhelmed. Simple matters become complex issues of great concern; discussions have to be faced where there is just not a viable answer to be found. Such problems need to be shared, listened to, acknowledged as important to the person concerned, and most important, recognized as unique. Life experience and maturity which leads 'a caring person' to say, for example, 'Oh yes, I know, I had the same problem with my husband', does not help the suffering person with his or her *own* problems. This is because the corollary of such a remark is: 'Oh if she coped, I ought to be able to too, so why can't I?' Thus the helping person has actually made the person in trouble feel worse. Guilt and inadequacy are added to anxiety.

I am therefore concerned with attempting to demonstrate in this chapter that social workers have a specific, not a peripheral part to play in the team approach to working with the terminally ill.

Terminal illness as loss

An individual and his family coping with terminal illness are facing loss of a dramatic and permanent kind. The ill person is facing loss of function, of finance through loss of employment availability, of independence, of control of himself and those around him, of his loved ones, as he faces death. The family are experiencing the same range of loss, augmented by fear of the future, fear of survival without the person they love. This clearly adds up to a very difficult time in the history of the family.

Some families have faced loss and crisis before – perhaps many times. It may be not the first time a death has occurred, possibly the family has faced redundancy, unemployment, ill health, moving etc. Such families are more likely to manage better, though it will depend on how the family have coped with previous loss. If they have come through the crisis letting themselves feel it, absorb it into their understanding of themselves, then they will be able to face the current trauma with some strength. If, however, the family have never faced a serious crisis before, or have not really coped with a previous one, then they are likely to be overwhelmed by current problems.

Mrs B was 29 when her husband was diagnosed as having terminal cancer. They had four children under the age of 10 and were living away from their country of origin, and so were isolated on the council estate where they were housed. At the time of Mr B's death, Mrs B expressed actively suicidal ideas, neglected the children, and in general was quite unable to cope. Over the next year she talked with me about the death of her mother, when Mrs B herself was 13. How she had had to take care of her father, until she escaped by marrying Mr B at 17 years of age; how they had come to England, where Mrs B then suffered a series of five miscarriages. Now at 29 years of age, her husband, whom she described as 'the best man in the world – totally devoted to his family', had also died.

In our conversations it was necessary to deal with the many losses in Mrs B's life, starting with the first, before we could look at the death of her husband. We needed to talk of the significance of each loss to Mrs B and how she had reacted, denying the problem because of her other responsibilities. How she was unable to 'carry on' this time, and how this inability to carry on had to happen if the compounded grief of many years was to be absorbed. Clearly the story is a long and complicated one.

Mrs B is now at the stage where she can consider her present position, and look at the possibilities open to her. She has made sense of her bereavements to the extent that she recognizes how they have made her the person she is today.

It would be a mistake for us to feel that Mrs B's story is unusual. Many people faced with a crisis today, shudder, thinking 'here we go again', and try to cope, to get through it, at great expense to their physical and emotional strength. Mrs B just had to let go at the particular time in her life when her husband died. It is our job to try and assess with the people we meet, what their reaction to loss might be, and how it can be shared and acknowledged.

The experience of grief

Commonly, families dealing with grief, either at the impending death of a member of the family, or at the actual death, will say that they feel ostracized by the community around. Neighbours, friends, even relatives are embarrassed, awkward, and say to themselves, 'Oh, I expect they want to be alone.' In fact, this is usually the last thing that people, either when anticipating bereavement, or when experiencing it, want. They need to talk about their loss, over and over again, because this is one way it becomes reality. They will be sad, tearful, withdrawn often, but greatly appreciate care extended by anyone coming to share the grief with them.

People usually stay away because they feel that such a weight of sadness must be a 'private thing' and that it is an intrusion to contact the bereaved person. This is usually a rationale for embarrassment and awkwardness. We feel we do not know what to do, so it would be better to do nothing; at all events, keep to a safe distance. Often a neighbour will cook a meal, but leave it on the doorstep. Contact must be avoided.

Grief is a private thing that we cannot understand. I am of course suggesting that the last sentence is not true. Bereavement is a particularly total form of loss, and loss is something we have all experienced, however trivial. The component parts are the same.

Stages of reaction to loss

Dr Elizabeth Kubler-Ross (1970) has identified what these component parts might be: denial, anger, depression, bargaining, acceptance. Such a list is not exhaustive, neither is loss experienced in such a tidy, catalogued way. However, when one is attempting to meet with another at their time of grief, it is useful to keep such a list in mind, to use as an indicator of what stage the person may have reached.

So, let us test the theory with an example of loss that most of us have experienced – having a tooth extracted! First there is the niggling pain of toothache, which persists as we *deny* its existence. We say, 'I must have eaten something particularly sweet', or 'I shouldn't eat ice cream after drinking tea' – anything to deny we have a bad tooth. Secondly comes the irritation, the *anger*: 'What a time for this to happen, I can't possibly fit in a trip to the dentist, they charge the earth', etc. Probably we'll be irritable with those around us, who wonder at our tetchiness so stay away. Next comes the *depression*: 'But I don't like going to the dentist, it hurts, my face will be swollen, I don't want to go, I just want to hide and go to bed with a hot water bottle!' Then the *bargaining*: 'Well, if I go to the dentist, I could just look in that dress shop next door, and perhaps buy that skirt I liked', or 'I deserve a treat if I go, that video centre is just along the road . . .' Finally *acceptance*: the dental appointment is made, it wasn't so bad as had been feared and the possibility of a future after the extraction can be considered. What was an overwhelming experience, dictating one's behaviour for a few days, has become an absorbed experience that can be accounted for.

Obviously the point is somewhat laboured, but important to understand. Grief at the death of a dearly loved person is experienced in just the same way as the toothache. And how much we wanted someone, everyone, to sympathize and share the horror of the toothache.

Having outlined briefly some of the processes experienced in bereavement, attention must be turned now to how it is that the caring team, and the social worker in particular, can help.

Practical issues

First there is a plethora of practical and material help to be offered. For the ill person and his family, probably the biggest problem is one of reduced finance. It is the social worker's job to advise on the range of benefits available to terminally ill people, especially when they are being cared for at home. Most of these benefits are handled by the Department of Health and Social Security (DHSS), and the particular ones I have found to be most applicable are:

1   Attendance Allowance – paid at a 12-hour or 24-hour rate to the ill person after a period of 6 months when requiring constant attention. Non-taxable and non-accountable for things like rent rebates.

2   Mobility Allowance – paid to people under retirement age who go out but are unable to use public transport. Again non-taxable and non-accountable.

3   Invalid Care Allowance – paid to members of a family (excluding a wife) who stay at home to give care. Only payable if not in receipt of other benefits.

4   Non-Contributory Invalidity Pension for Married Women – payable to ill married women who paid National Insurance contributions at women's rate only when they were working, and so are not eligible for sickness benefit. This benefit is taken into account when assessing any other family member's benefit, e.g. unemployment, supplementary, and sickness benefit.

Most of these are payable for up to 4 weeks of a patient's hospitalization. Most of the pensions, e.g. retirement, are reduced after an 8-week stay in hospital, and the relevant DHSS office should always be informed when a patient in receipt of benefit or pension is admitted to hospital. A person in receipt of supplementary benefit is entitled to have visiting fares to hospital paid. However, the circumstances of each individual always have to be looked at when trying to discuss what benefits will be most suitable for the person concerned.

Additionally it is often possible to contact national charities on the family's behalf. Amongst these the National Society for Cancer Relief is probably the most pertinent and certainly very generous and helpful! It helps in two ways: first with a special grant for a particular need, such as an outstanding heating bill or travelling fares for treatment, a holiday etc.; secondly with a regular weekly grant to help towards the increased cost of caring for a seriously ill person, again especially at home. Another charity to contact is the Malcolm Sargent Cancer Fund, which helps with the financial need of families where there is an ill child.

A family is coping with the trauma of terminal disease, the last thing it should have to be concerned about is financial stress, and a considerable amount can be done to alleviate this. When the ward staff notice that a patient isn't being visited regularly by his family, how often is it considered that the cost of travelling might be prohibitive? As a family realizes that one of its members has a limited time left, often there emerges a particular aspiration, a goal that needs to be met. It is often the social worker's task to discuss this and help it to become reality. For example, my recent caseload has included: central heating installed before a father died; a flat redecorated; rehousing; visiting family members in another country; making a will and provision for the family; restoring relationships with long-estranged relatives; and very often getting a telephone installed quickly.

There are an increasing number of patients referred with prescribed industrial disease, and then it is important to arrange claims for industrial disease benefit; a complicated and protracted business. The Society for Prevention of Asbestosis and Industrial Disease (SPAID), a national self-help organization established to put such people in touch with each other, is immensely helpful in negotiating this process.

After the patient has died the practical involvement continues. Quite often families will need help with arranging the actual funeral. Again finance is often a real problem, and families may need advice about 'public funerals' and the resources of the DHSS, if families are receiving supplementary benefit. Following that, dealing with probate, widow's allowances and pensions, building societies for rearranging mortgages etc. all needs to be done. Widows often need help with disposing of the car, finding the gas and electricity meters, even how to get on a bus, which hitherto had never been done alone. Widowers ask for help with simple cooking recipes, the mysteries of the launderette and supermarket.

It might be thought that the preceding paragraph represents a stereotype view of the traditional sex roles in British society which is fast becoming irrelevant. In my experience that is still, regrettably, just not so. For the vast majority of people in the younger as well as the older age group, a man moves straight from his parent's home to his marital home, and has no experience of living on his own, learning the range of tasks traditionally performed by the opposite sex!

Other areas of help

Social workers give considerable emotional support to patients and their families. The social worker will often be the only non-medical member of the terminal care team, and this is an important aspect to emphasize.

It is by no means the social worker's lone task to be listening to the patient and his family: the whole team is involved in this; but the social worker will often be chosen by the family to express their doubts and worries to, precisely because of this obvious non-medical presentation. However caring and considerate the medical members of the team, families are often embarrassed to ask what they imagine might be stupid questions. It is easier to ask a lay person such as themselves. I well remember a lady at home looking at me in a puzzled way, and asking how she was supposed to administer suppositories to herself in what was clearly an anatomically impossible position. Once I explained, with many giggles, the cause of Mrs F's continuing and puzzling constipation became clear! She had felt she could not ask the nurse for instructions and so had been administering them as directed. Indeed she had been, but not in the relevant orifice!

The same sort of approach is needed for discussion on diagnosis, prognosis etc. Working in a traditional medical social work setting, the social worker is usually very limited in what she is able to discuss with the family. Working as an integrated team and ward member she is as intrinsically involved in this as any other team member.

Again the family may well choose to ask the social worker their deepest questions. Often it is the social worker who is seen to have more time, unencumbered by nursing procedures, and in general is more often asked to explain in language the family understands.

As has been previously discussed, the social worker is centrally involved in helping a patient who has become overwhelmed by his impending loss of life. Referring back to the stages of loss, some patients will deny their illness to a disabling degree, so that no honest communication can be carried out by the family at all. Others will become extremely embittered – constantly asking 'Why me?' – and remain there, instead of moving along the spectrum to a 'well, I don't like it but I accept it' attitude. In my experience it is more likely to be the family denying what is happening, than the patient.

Miss D, a patient living with an elderly mother, resolutely refused to agree that anything was worrying her at all. She would soon recover from this 'virus' and then continue to look after her mother. She became very angry and distressed as we tried to discuss with her the fact that her level of obvious anxiety must be connected to concern for herself: 'No, it's not, it's you who upset me,' she would say, and then would plaintively add, 'you must be able to do something to make me better.'

The most usual situation is that the family need to be reassured that nothing catastrophic will happen if they discuss diagnosis with their relative. Often the patient has already conveyed to the team that 'he knows', but he is afraid to talk it over with the family, who 'won't be able to take it'. The family have conveyed exactly the same thing! What a tragedy that conspiracy and counter-plot should enter a family's history at this stage, especially if there has always been open communication before. It becomes the social worker's job to explain to both parties, that the other is waiting to talk things over, and that no one will collapse. What a difference open communication can make, and in bereavement follow-up work the family will always remind me of that particular conversation. They remember with absolute clarity how it came about, and with thanksgiving that it did.

A sizeable proportion of patients, however, are alone in the world, and as such need the team to become their 'family'.

Follow-up care

Bereavement follow-up is again a team task, if possible, not just the social worker's. It is essential to convey the conviction that the whole team is concerned for the whole family, not just the patient. They come to us at a vulnerable time in their development as a family. This is a privilege and a responsibility that needs to be recognized. However, it is often the social worker who has most contact with the family, by nature of the tasks we cover.

When making a home visit, I am often immediately whisked into the kitchen, without catching sight of the patient, to discuss the family's worries. Their fears of not coping, their anxieties about how death will come, how they will manage, what they will do – their worries sometimes seem endless. There is often only a final and cursory 'Did you call to see my husband/wife/mother?'. This seems to me to be entirely appropriate, and for this reason much of the bereavement follow-up work comes the social worker's way.

The emotional vulnerability of grieving people is well documented. The surviving relative, especially if old, young, isolated or weighed down by other worries is highly likely to become ill, have an accident or a breakdown, and in not a few instances die soon after bereavement. Suicide is a real risk for some people, with the survivor feeling that life is totally meaningless and just cannot be tolerated. Generalizations are of limited use, but usually we would be involved with a relative whom we consider to be at risk in this way for approximately 15 months.

Immediately following the death of the loved relative, the survivor is surrounded by activity. There is a great deal to arrange, numerous relatives arrive. Often the survivor quickly takes a holiday, stays with relatives, returns to work, becomes absorbed in activity of some sort or another. This may be necessary, but it usually has the effect of extending the first stage of grief, i.e. denial. After this stage of activity, the survivor finds him/herself one day sitting alone in the home that had been shared, and feels a desolation and aloneness that is quite shattering. Some respond by feeling they must move, change jobs, do something, but this is seldom helpful. There are no short cuts through grief, which is why the sharing of it with a trusted friend can be so vital.

I find it of infinite worth that I knew the family before the death of the patient, because often I can become that friend for a period of time: to talk through, as often as it takes, what has happened, and how. The qualities of the deceased person are pondered and, especially important, what the surviving relative did to care for the loved one. It greatly aids the grieving process if the relative is able to say realistically, 'I did everything I could to look after him/her.' Many relatives who have had to have their loved person hospitalized will feel guilty that they did so, however impossible any other alternative was.

A timely word of caution is appropriate here. Many relationships are not totally loving. (Such a statement will not surprise the reader, I am sure.) Some families take care of a sick relative for many motives other than selfless loving, and it is no part of a social worker's job to judge what the motives might be. It is, however, important to understand and listen to what they are, because they can crucially affect the grieving process. For some survivors, the overwhelming feeling is of relief.

Mrs T had been a 'battered wife' for 8 years, and although her husband was very considerably weakened by his terminal illness, she was still in great fear of him. Mrs T nursed her husband motivated by this fear, not by care, and she unhappily confessed to me that she was praying for a release from this torment by her husband's death. The complex emotions that follow on through a bereavement of this kind need careful handling.

It is an old adage 'don't speak ill of the dead', and when an individual such as Mrs T feels she has somehow willed the death to happen, the future life that she thought would be a releasing one quickly turns to a guilt-ridden one.

Gradually the year of bereavement continues. The first Christmas, birthday, wedding anniversary, and eventually the anniversary of the death, are important milestones; generally very sad ones. Hospices usually send a card to the family on the anniversary of the patient's death, saying simply that the staff are thinking of the family on a difficult day. If it is known that the surviving relative is going to be alone on that day, personal contact will be attempted.

After this crucial first anniversary when the bereaved person can begin to realize it is no longer 'this time last year' but 'this time the year before', the raw grief gives way to an absorbed sadness that of course still hurts, but is more likely to be seen as part of life's dealings; and it is at this time that the special work task may be complete. There is still the need for follow-up support home care which may well be provided by Cruse, a national organization for widows and widowers, or by the Society of Compassionate Friends, an organization for parents who have had a child die. Unfortunately such groups are in short supply, especially in inner-city areas. Bereavement counselling services are beginning to grow, and referral to them may be entirely appropriate. Friendships are made, grieving people realize they are not alone in feeling as they do, and that is an important step along the bereavement process.

The social worker as a team member

The particular kind of social work that I have tried to describe – in a terminal care team – is a demanding one, and all the team's members find it so. As the social worker, one is often called upon to listen to other members of the team, and to share the concerns that such a demanding job can produce. This seems to me to be an entirely valid social work activity. We are perhaps uniquely qualified amongst the health care team to understand something of the way pressures can distress and overwhelm a colleague, however experienced he or she may be. As I have tried to suggest, we may often not be so actively involved in the primary symptom control function of the team. What we are available for, is to talk with the team members who are so involved, recognizing the need for such work to be constantly reviewed and assessed.

Reference

Kubler-Ross, E (1970) On Death and Dying, Tavistock

CHAPTER 14

THE ROLE OF VARIOUS THERAPISTS
SISTER MARY WYNNE and MARION JUDD

THE PLACE OF CREATIVE AND DIVERSIONAL ACTIVITIES
Sister Mary Wynne

To be creative and useful is a necessity for every human being. Those who are terminally ill, as well as the handicapped and the disabled, are not exempt from this necessity and need to prove that they can still be useful and creative. This need should be encouraged as far as possible and such people should not be made to feel that 'they are pushed to the margins of society', to quote the words of Pope John Paul II.

Uses of a centre for creative activities

Any institution caring for the dying should be provided with a suitably equipped centre for the purpose of helping terminally ill patients to find an occupation which is of interest to them as individuals and which they can enjoy. The centre could also be used by patients who are being nursed at home, if they are able to be brought to it without causing them too much effort or strain. (It might be possible for a domiciliary therapist to visit patients at home if or when they cannot get to the centre.)

It is important to remember that there are many stages and degrees of severity in terminal illness and that each case must be treated individually, so that the therapy is used to maximum effect.

Although a nucleus of trained staff is desirable, many volunteers can be used to assist in the various activities. Those specially trained in arts and crafts can guide the patients whose function may be limited in several ways, so that they have the satisfaction of achieving something, however small.

It is much better to begin with a simple occupation which can be completed rather than undertake a too ambitious task which is beyond the ability of an individual. Personal tastes must also be considered and one may have to persevere with a variety of suggestions before one finds the occupation congenial to a particular person. Latent talents often appear even at the late stage of an illness, which may amaze relatives and sometimes even the patient himself.

No pressure must be placed on any patient: he must feel free to come to the centre if and when he chooses and stay away without being made to feel that he is upsetting anyone.

Gardening activities If the centre has a garden this is an added attraction, as many terminally ill patients get real pleasure from just sitting and enjoying the colours, sounds and scents around them, and the changes that occur with the seasons; or they may get simple delight from feeding the birds or doing a little light gardening, especially if this has been a hobby of theirs in the past.

Musical activities Listening to music is another pastime which the dying patient may enjoy: radio or cassettes may be used and the patient's special favourites provided for him. Some may like to play the piano, even if only for a short time, and at Christmas-tide carols are often sung, giving immense pleasure to many. Local community groups sometimes offer to entertain patients with concerts or short plays, and provided the entertainment is not too long, these groups are to be welcomed.

Diversional activities Patients who are regular Bingo enthusiasts may continue to play if they wish, and there are plenty of other games, puzzles and simple competitions to keep them entertained. Cards, jigsaws, quizzes, word games, such as crossword or Scrabble, should all be available to provide interest and entertainment for all tastes. Some of these are more suitable for patients who, though physically affected, are still mentally active, but all patients should be encouraged to find a diversional activity which they can enjoy. Painting, drawing or sculpture may be an ideal relaxation for some.

Library Use can be made of books with large print and talking books for those who find difficulty using ordinary books.

Visitors

Frequent short visits from relatives and friends give immense pleasure, but the nurse in charge must make sure that visitors do not overtire the patient by staying too long or pouring out their own troubles.

Chatting to someone about his interests is good for the patient and he may like the visitor to help him finish the crossword or jigsaw puzzle he has begun. Nurses do not always realize how tiring it is for patients to make the effort to talk to their visitors, so they should observe the patient and if they notice any signs of strain, they should tactfully suggest that the visitors return again later. Close relatives must be given priority at the bedside and here again tact is required if neighbours or casual friends are tending to monopolize the patient's attention.

Children give great pleasure and happiness by their presence in a ward or in the patient's home. Obviously noisy, boisterous behaviour would be tiring, but a short time spent at the bedside provides a welcome diversion for the patient. (Space should be available for the children then to play within view of the family.)

A dying patient in a hospice or hospital may suddenly express a longing to visit his home again, realizing, perhaps, that this is for the last time. Every effort should be made to meet this request even though it may be considered rather a hazardous undertaking. Neighbours and friends will usually be only too willing to assist the family with transport and help with lifting or carrying the patient within his home.

Social occasions

There may be some important family event, such as a daughter's wedding, when the patient literally stays alive long enough to achieve this desire of attending, and then 'lets go' contentedly. Small social gatherings should be encouraged: family and friends gathered round the patient to mark a birthday or to show off a new baby. A few moments at a time may be enough, or longer if the patient is obviously enjoying the company.

Memories of occasions such as these will be precious to the family when the time comes to sit with their dying relative at the end, no longer able to respond and share in their thoughts and activities.

HOW PHYSIOTHERAPY CAN HELP THE DYING PATIENT
Marion Judd

When a person is dying, those who are looking after him, both medical staff and family, may feel that physiotherapy is inappropriate. However, if the aim of the terminal care team is to maintain the best quality of life possible for that patient, physiotherapy has certain things to offer to further that aim. The role of physiotherapy in this field is not only palliative, but has an active contribution to make towards symptom control. Furthermore, physiotherapy is closely concerned with rehabilitation, which is often possible and indeed desirable in the terminally ill, as one's concern must be for enhancing the quality of life wherever practicable, and thus enabling the patient to do the things he wants to. A patient can be helped far more to come to terms with his condition if his physical symptoms can be controlled and the physiotherapist's place in the sympton control team can thus be positively justified.

Pain

Now that pain control techniques by medication are so greatly improved, good pain control can be achieved by drugs alone in a great many cases, providing the patient has faith in his physician. However, there are some instances where the use of physiotherapy treatment is indicated to augment the medication. Just to mention the stiff and painful joints which rapidly occur in the paraplegic or hemiparetic patient and which can be prevented or alleviated by regular passive movements will suffice. Also any pre-existing condition which is present alongside a malignant disease, and which requires physiotherapy treatment, normally can still be treated with benefit to the patient.

The usual physiotherapy treatments using heat, ice, ultrasound and exercises need to be borne in mind. A new modality for the control of pain is the transcutaneous nerve stimulator (TNS). Much work is currently being done on its use in this country and we should see physiotherapists using it much more in the future. It has been found to be valuable in the relief of pain caused by nerve root compression. It also gives excellent pain relief in herpes zoster, which is sometimes found in patients with malignant disease. Future developments in this field of pain relief should be watched for. Acupuncture also is a treatment modality used by some physiotherapists and there is increasing interest in its effects. Acupuncture may well be found to have a place in the management of pain by physical means in the future.

Oedema

In the oedematous limb where there is partial obstruction of venous or lymphatic drainage, the physiotherapist can help relieve symptoms by using a Jobst pump. This gives intermittent pressure to the whole limb and helps to drain it. When it is combined with a regime of elevation and gentle exercises the discomfort is lessened and there is improvement of function and cosmetic effect.

Stiffness

There are very many causes of stiffness but in the terminally ill patient who may have been bedridden for a considerable time the joints can easily become stiff. It is important to maintain as full a range of joint movement as possible, first to prevent discomfort and improve function, and secondly to make nursing care easier. The physiotherapist can give passive and active movements to all joints as a preventive measure.

Loss of mobility

Often the physiotherapist is called in to treat a patient who, after months of pain and immobility, has had his pain controlled. These patients can sometimes be mobilized, i.e. helped to walk about again, climb stairs, get on and off chairs and toilet seats and in and out of bed. Progressive exercises are given to mobilize joints and strengthen muscles. Practice is given in regaining lost skills as strength returns. The home situation is taken into account in regaining mobility, as there may be stairs to relearn to negotiate, small toilets to manoeuvre in and out of, awkward corners to turn, and difficulty in getting in and out of the bath to overcome. The strengthening and mobilization of the arms will help the patient to dress, wash himself and do his hair, reach up to light switches and cupboards etc., and achieve more independence in his activities of daily living. Appropriate walking aids are provided and advice on suitable footwear given. If such things as shoe build-ups are required, the physiotherapist can assess and arrange for their provision.

Splinting

Appropriate splinting can add to a patient's comfort. Perhaps a collar is needed to support a painful neck or a splint to support a hand or foot. The physiotherapist can either make these or arrange to have them made.

Chest conditions

The dying patient is prone to chest infections. He may also be a chronic bronchitic or have asthma. Physiotherapy for these latter conditions can be given routinely if the patient is relatively well, i.e. nebulized salbutamol and breathing exercises, percussion and vibrations. There is a time when it is inappropriate to treat the patient, when no further advantage can be gained from active treatment, but there is also a time when assistance in clearing secretions will be helpful in relieving the persistent coughing and dyspnoea which is so exhausting to a weak and ill patient. If the secretions are profuse some gentle percussion and vibrations can be given. Steam inhalations and relaxation techniques also have their place. The physical contact from the physiotherapist can provide comfort and reassurance even if only a very little actual treatment is possible.

Teaching

The physiotherapist has a teaching role, especially in home care. She is able to show families how to lift patients; give advice on positioning for comfort or chest drainage; show families how best to help the patient walk, get on and off chairs and in and out of baths, and transfer from bed to chair etc. Often the physiotherapist will need to call on occupational therapy colleagues who can advise and provide aids and adaptations in the home to increase the patient's ability to function independently.

Listening

A patient may choose to discuss his problems with any member of the caring team. Often, when he is having physical treatment, the physiotherapist will hear about matters which concern the patient deeply, and as part of the team, she is able to make sure that suitable professional help is offered to him. In this time of family crisis there is a need for careful and patient listening, and the whole team has to be very well aware of the roles of other disciplines so that problems can be dealt with by the appropriate person.

The multidisciplinary team approach needed to cater for the physical, mental and spiritual needs of the dying patient has a place for the physiotherapist therefore, not only wearing the traditional rehabilitative hat, but also giving a positive contribution to symptom control.

Reference

Downie, P A (1978) Cancer Rehabilitation – An introduction for physiotherapists and the allied professions, Faber and Faber

CHAPTER 15

RELIGIOUS BELIEFS AND PRACTICES
REVEREND PAUL McGINN and
JOY ROBBINS

Many dying people will find considerable support from a religious system of faith and worship which has been an important background to their lives, even if only practised intermittently. Ministers of religion should therefore be accepted as colleagues by members of the caring team. The term 'minister' is apt, meaning one who brings aid and gives a service; but, of course, various titles will be used -- priest, vicar, rabbi, imam --and it is courteous to discover the acceptable title and use it in each case.

Where there is anxiety on the part of the family that their dying relative should be kept in ignorance of his condition, the view may be expressed that a visit from a minister may be upsetting and arouse suspicion in the patient's mind. Apart from other considerations, it can be pointed out that patients are used to seeing clergymen of various denominations in a hospital ward. Both here and in the patient's own home his wishes must be of paramount concern, and the nurse should acquaint the particular minister with the situation if the family has not done so.

The nurse's attitude

In respecting the patient's right to practise his own religious beliefs, assistance should readily be given to his religious minister. This requires a basic knowledge of what will be needed for any special rites and ceremonies. In his turn, the minister will be anxious to co-operate with staff and often only needs to be escorted to the patient and afforded some privacy such as drawing the bed curtains. Sometimes, unfortunately, a minister will only be asked to come at a very late stage in the final illness, rather than earlier when he can be of great comfort to the patient and family, continuing to help the latter during the period of bereavement.

Christian ministries

In this country at the present time, the nurse will meet patients belonging to many different Christian denominations, differing in certain beliefs and practices but united in a common faith in Jesus Christ and in a life after death. Each denomination will have a particular form of caring for its members when they are dying, and examples of this from the main Christian groups are given here.

The Anglican Communion

The Church of England offers a number of rites for assisting the dying person. The Book of Common Prayer in the order for the visitation of the sick directs the priest to establish with the patient:

1   Penitence – sorrow for wrongdoing.
2   Charity – by restoring relationships, making a will, settling debts.
3   Increase of the sick person's faith.

These basic pastoral aims will be met in the way that is appropriate and helpful for the individual. There is a rite of anointing, as in the Roman Catholic Church, and provision for confession of his sins to a priest, if the person wishes, and to receive Holy Communion. Many Anglicans find their greatest comfort in readings of the Scriptures and in prayer. At the moment of death, special Commendatory prayers may be said by the priest or those caring for the patient, including members of the family.

The Roman Catholic Church

There are a number of Sacraments and rites laid down for the spiritual comfort of the dying Catholic and his family.

The Sacrament of Penance and Reconciliation   This is popularly known as 'Confession'. Any person who expresses in some way a wish to receive this Sacrament should be left alone with the priest. The person is reminded that God is a God of love and mercy and he is invited to acknowledge his past sins and his sorrow for them. The words of forgiveness ('absolution') are spoken by the priest on behalf of the Church and are an assurance of complete forgiveness by a loving Saviour. It is not necessary for the patient to be able to speak – the priest will probably be able to ascertain the person's dispositions. For some 'Confession' will have been a regular feature throughout their life; for others, along with other traditional Catholic practices, there well may have been a period of lapsing.

The Sacrament of the Sick   This Sacrament is offered to those whose illness gives cause for concern. Formerly known as 'Last Rites', the original name (Sacrament of the Sick) has been restored to emphasize that in terms of faith it is a source of strength and consolation for the sick person. Whereas the Sacrament of Penance will normally be a private encounter between patient and priest, the Church encourages others to be present at the Sacrament of the Sick, especially members of the family and those caring for the patient. In this way the concern of the Church will be expressed as a communal concern and the patient will be aware of the prayers offered for him by all. There will be times when the presence of others is not feasible. During this Sacrament a passage from Scripture is read (usually one of the healing episodes in the life of Jesus), prayers for the person are said, and after the priest has laid his hands on the head of the patient in silence, he anoints the patient's forehead and palms of the hands with holy oil and says the accompanying prayers.

The Sacrament of Holy Communion   In this Sacrament a passage from Scripture may be read, the Lord's Prayer said, and Communion given, followed by a prayer and blessing. If it is obvious that this may be the last time the patient can receive, special prayers are said to commend him on his last journey.

Prayers for the Dying Person   When death is near there are certain prayers and readings which can be said for the dying person and for the comfort and consolation of those close by. If the priest is not present (and it is not necessary for him to be if the Sacraments mentioned above have already been administered) then the prayers may be read by anyone present.

Free Churches

These comprise the third main Christian group in this country, and share many common beliefs with each other, and with the Anglican and Catholic communities. For the purposes of this chapter, the nurse will find that members of these Churches share with other Christians hope for a life after death, and that dying patients and their families will look for comfort and spiritual help from their ministers. There are no special rites practised, but an emphasis on the mercy of God, and inspiration from Scripture readings and spontaneous prayers together. Congregations of the various Free Churches are noted for being close-knit communities with a caring attitude to those in need, including their own members.

Non-Christian Religions

Rituals associated with dying and death are often closely associated with religion. Patients of cultures other than the Western model may profess a non-Christian religion, with implications for physical care as well as religious observance. Some information in this respect is provided here of four of the major non-Christian religions. The reader is referred to more detailed studies in the list of references at the end of this chapter.

Judaism

The patient may belong to either the Liberal or Orthodox category of Judaism. In the case of the former there will be few special requirements, although some Liberal Jews will observe strict rules concerning their diet, which will be either vegetarian or kosher (i.e. meat must come from animals slaughtered in a special way, and any meat from the pig is forbidden). There are no formal last rites, but prayers for the dying may be said by the rabbi or family and friends. The Orthodox Jew follows a number of strict rules regarding daily living. In particular, he will eat only a kosher diet, and any food or drugs which come from the pig are forbidden. The dying person will wish the rabbi to be with him in his last hours to help him acknowledge his sins and to recite special prayers.

When carrying out Last Offices the nurse can only close the eyes, straighten the limbs and bandage the jaw. The body is then transferred to the mortuary where a member of the synagogue or family will be in attendance. The body will then be washed by specially trained officials from the local Jewish burial society.

Islam

The religion of Islam is followed by Muslims. Every day a Muslim should pray to Allah (God) at least five times, and before prayers will perform special ablutions. Nurses should be aware of the reluctance of some Muslim women to be undressed or examined in the presence of a man other than their husband. Muslims do not eat any food which comes from the pig, and fast at the festival of Ramadan, although the seriously ill person will be dispensed from this.

There is no equivalent to the Christian priest or Jewish rabbi, but the religious teacher is known as the Imam. He may be asked to visit the dying patient; otherwise the family will recite prayers in Arabic; the patient must face Mecca while doing so. (In Britain this means that the feet will be pointing to the south-east.)

After death the body is washed by members of the family, and will then be placed in special pieces of cloth. The Muslim family will wish the burial to take place as quickly as possible, a coffin not being acceptable. Help and advice regarding these matters can be obtained from the Muslim Information Centre, or from the nearest Islamic Centre.

Hinduism

Hinduism has no fixed creed and many schools of philosophical thought. Hindus practise polytheism (worship of many gods and godesses). As with Muslim women, the nurse will find that Hindu women dislike, and may refuse, examination by a male doctor. A practising Hindu will not eat food that comes from cattle, believing that the cow is a sacred animal. The dying patient's family may wish to remain at the bedside, especially the eldest son, even if only a small child. The local Hindu priest – the Pundit – may come to pray with the patient and read passages from the holy books. After death, relatives will wash the body and dress it in new clothes. The husband of a deceased Hindu woman cuts the marriage thread placed round her neck at marriage – no-one else may do this.

Buddhism

Buddhist teaching is based on non-violence and brotherhood, and on reincarnation. There are no special aspects of care except that some Buddhists are vegetarian. The practice of meditation is important at certain times of the day, and the patient may like to have a small statue of Buddha with him. There are no special rites for the dying but the patient and his family may wish to be visited by a Buddhist monk.

It should be realized that followers of these religions originate from countries where family ties are close, and this tendency continues if migration to another country such as Britain occurs. It is thus understandable that a number of relatives may congregate together round the dying patient's bed and that outward signs of grief will be manifested to an extent which may be disturbing to other patients in a hospital ward. In this situation the nurse should be ready to escort the relatives to a suitable room after the death has taken place so that they may support each other and give vent to their grief in private. Because of the close-knit family circle there is usually considerable support during bereavement from within the family and close friends of the deceased.

The nurse may meet patients from many other religious faiths than those mentioned. It is helpful if clear guidelines are available in patient areas regarding telephone numbers of religious centres where the appropriate minister can be contacted; and if some notes are drawn up for nurses with details of any religious practices which are important to patients when they are gravely ill.

Bereavement

Even for those with no formal religious beliefs, a clergyman together with doctors and nurses represents a service offered to their dying relative, and to themselves at the time. After the death, the minister of religion with the funeral director is accepted as having a rightful function to perform in aiding the living to accept the final separation from the dead person.

The family who has seen the minister bringing comfort to their dying relative will often turn for support themselves before and after the death, and ask for help in making decisions such as whether to allow children to attend the funeral.

The funeral is a very important event as the culmination of a process of care for the dying and bereaved, although care for the latter must go on. Rituals allow human beings to express feelings collectively which can be difficult to express openly and completely as individuals. Thus, the funeral rite is one way of enabling the bereaved to feel 'allowed' to grieve.

The role of the minister, in arranging the funeral as the relatives wish, in visiting them before and afterwards, and in leading the community in open recognition of the reality of the final separation of death, is crucial. The minister, as leader of his local church, will also ensure that the community shares with him the task of continuing to support the bereaved member of the congregation in appropriate ways, especially in offering to visit.

References

Ainsworth-Smith, I and Speck, P (1982) Letting Go – Caring for the Dying and Bereaved, SPCK

Hector, W. and Whitfield, S (1982) Nursing Care for the Dying Patient and the Family, Heinemann Medical

Hinton, J (1972) Dying, Pelican

Lamerton, R (1981) Care of the Dying, Pelican

Sampson, C (1982) The Neglected Ethic, McGraw Hill

Zaechner, R C (1971) The Concise Encyclopedia of Living Faiths, 2nd edition, Hutchinson

CHAPTER 16

ETHICAL ASPECTS
JOY ROBBINS*

Ethics is the scientific and philosophical study which seeks to determine and to provide guidance towards goodness in human actions. Ethical principles are meant to provide a basis for everyday practice and all professions establish their own ethical codes for their members to follow.

Involvement with death and dying poses many ethical problems and dilemmas. Life itself is a person's most valuable possession, and the duty to preserve human life is upheld in the ethical codes of both the nursing and medical professions. Difficulties can arise in the interpretation of principles and their application to the actual situation when the doctor or nurse often has to make decisions in a short space of time. Sometimes two professional people will come to different conclusions about an ethical dilemma even though both have given serious and sincere thought to the problem. Cultural and religious factors can influence a person deeply in coming to a decision.

Examples of ethical dilemmas associated with death and dying

Use of powerful opiate or sedative drugs
The principle of relieving pain and distress in the dying patient is

---

*I wish to acknowledge the help of Dr R Corcoran in writing this chapter.

honourable and humanitarian, and administration of drugs where a proper regime is used should be uncontroversial (see Chapter 6). An anxiety is sometimes expressed that a nurse does not wish to be the one to give 'the last injection', implying that it is this which will kill the patient. This is erroneous; the patient having pain control management as described dies of his disease, not from the drugs.

The opposite situation may occur where the nurse considers that a patient is receiving inadequate analgesia and is in pain, but the doctor is reluctant to alter the medication. Consulting with a more senior nursing colleague and both discussing the matter with the doctor are the appropriate steps to take to resolve the problem.

The patient's rights

In endeavouring to act in the best interests of the patient, the caring team must be careful to include his views as far as possible. The patient's rights have also to be balanced with those of others. For instance, a patient may wish to die at home but despite all the help that could be arranged it would create an overwhelming problem for the family. In this case it would not be right to press the issue even though it means overriding the patient's wishes. The patient has a right to know about his illness and prognosis insofar as he wishes to do so. From the right to know follows a further right – to refuse active treatment. In the dying patient with advancing cancer this could arise in relation to an option of further radiotherapy being given. Occasionally a patient may refuse to take drugs being given for symptom control. These rights must be respected by the care-givers, having ensured that the patient has had the situation fully discussed with him and that he understands any consequences likely to follow his refusal. If a patient is not lucid, then such decisions must be made for him.

Resuscitation and use of life-support systems

In a general hospital it is often a student nurse who initiates resuscitation in a patient who suddenly suffers a cardiac arrest. Clear guidance is essential in the ward as to when resuscitation should be carried out, and which patients this is inappropriate for. The staff should understand why particular decisions are made. Good communication will remove uncertainty and worry that the 'wrong' action has been taken.

Nurses will be very involved in the care of a patient whose vital functions are being maintained by a life-support system. If it is thought to be no longer reasonable to continue ventilation of the patient since brain death has been confirmed, the medical staff in charge should discuss the matter with the family and with the whole caring team before the machine is switched off. This is a traumatic situation for all concerned, and it should be made clear that this is not a case of killing a patient, because he is already dead.

Maintenance of fluid and nutrition in dying patients

This is not only a practical but an emotive issue. Next to the need for oxygen, the needs for water and then food are universally recognized as the fundamental drives to maintain life. If during the terminal illness a person is unable to eat or drink normally, decisions must be taken by his carers as to the proper course of action. Those most involved hitherto will have been nurses and the patient's family, particularly if he is at home. Once normal intake becomes impossible, the management of the situation involves others to a greater extent, especially the doctor and dietitian.

There is no single answer to the problem, each person must be assessed individually and his entire circumstances taken into account. This is again a situation in which the patient should be included in the decision making if possible. One of the following options will be available:

1   If the patient is considered to be deteriorating rapidly, becoming semiconscious and likely to die within about 48 hours, no artificial feeding will be instituted but the patient's mouth will be kept moist.

2   A problem may arise when it is judged that the patient, although in the terminal stage of his illness, has still several weeks to live. An example is the patient with advanced carcinoma of oesophagus who is now having difficulty even with swallowing liquids. It might be considered right to attempt to pass a fine-bore nasogastric tube and institute tube feeding, or to commence an intravenous infusion of a suitable fluid. However, the patient and the team together may decide that he should not have this artificial treatment as this would only be an additional burden in his process of dying. Every means would be taken to ensure the patient's comfort and tranquillity, including medication and constant mouth care.

3   A patient may be admitted for terminal care to hospital or hospice, or transferred home from hospital, with some means of artificial feeding

already in place. This might include a gastrostomy. Unless there is some problem actually being caused by the feeding apparatus itself, the decision is likely to be that the feeding should continue until circumstances change.

4   There has been much publicity recently about attitudes towards newborn handicapped infants. Debate centres on how the rights of such children to proper care, including ordinary provision of fluid and nutrition, should be met within the particular circumstances. Such decisions involve the parents, and doctors and nurses who have accepted responsibility for doing their best in the interests of the patient and the family. Nurses cannot opt out in such decision making, particularly as the patient is unable to speak for himself. One of the basic principles of nursing care is to help the patient with eating and drinking. The same ethical principles should be applied to care of the infant human being as to adults, whether the child is handicapped or not. If this is not so, the question must be asked, whether a mental or physical handicap renders a person subhuman. If the newborn infant is dying, any decision regarding whether or not some means of artificial feeding should be attempted must, as in the case of adults, be taken in the light of all the prevailing circumstances.

Rights of the nurse

If the nurse is asked to carry out or participate in some treatment which she is convinced is unethical, she has the right to refuse to do so. It is important that such a step is only taken when the nurse is sure that she has full and accurate knowledge and understanding of the situation, and that by withdrawing she does not harm the patient in another way. An example would be where a nurse is working in an operating theatre and suddenly refuses on ethical grounds to assist the surgeon who is performing an abortion. If the patient bleeds severely the nurse would be held gravely at fault if she did not remain during this crisis and give assistance. The law provides a disassociation clause for non-participation in abortions and the nurse should have made her position clear to the theatre superintendent well in advance.

Euthanasia

This Greek word literally means 'a good death'. It is the modern interpretation (popularly 'mercy killing') of the word which has given rise to frequent and continuing debate at least since 1936 with the founding of the Euthanasia Society, in 1969 changing its name to the Voluntary Euthanasia Society and now known as EXIT.

Euthanasia now means in practice:

> deliberately bring about the death of a human being on the grounds of certain factors regarding the quality of his life now and in the future, and sometimes that of his family.

The majority of doctors and nurses are opposed to euthanasia, although there is a small but increasing pressure group in society at large who uphold the concept in certain circumstances. Not only ethical reasons but the foreseeable consequences for themselves should euthanasia be legalized account for the opposition of the medical and nursing professions. They would be directly involved as the providers and sometimes the administrators of lethal doses of drugs. The arguments for and against euthanasia can easily be found elsewhere and will not be discussed further here except for one point. Those who oppose euthanasia should be in the forefront in helping to provide high standards of care for the dying, the handicapped and the despairing members of society. 'It seems a terrible indictment that the main argument for euthanasia is that many suffer unduly because there is a lack of preparation and provision for the total care of the dying.' (Hinton 1972). The same statement could be made of the other groups for whom euthanasia is advocated as a solution to their sufferings.

Conclusion

The ethical dimensions of modern medicine pose many difficult problems for the nurse, and the challenge must be met by becoming as well informed as possible regarding the principles involved. In coming to what is regarded as the right decision, experience, intelligent reasoning and desire to uphold the patient's interests all contribute. Religious convictions do not necessarily make the pathway easier but do provide an added meaning to matters of life and death. In disagreeing with others, one should respect the individual for sincerely held views, and be aware of the personal anguish that ethical problems often bring to those involved.

This chapter has been written in the light of traditional Christian principles upheld by the author, and applied to the care of dying patients in the hospice where she works.

References

Dunstan, G R (1978) Discerning the duties, in C M Saunders (Editor) The Management of Terminal Disease, Edward Arnold

Hector, W and Whitfield, S (1982) Nursing Care for the Dying Patient and the Family, William Heinemann Medical Books

Henderson, V (1969) Basic Principles of Nursing Care, International Council of Nurses

Hinton, J (1972) Dying, Pelican Books

Lamerton, R (1980) Care of the Dying, Pelican Books

Linacre Centre, The (1982) Euthanasia and Clinical Practice – Trends, principles and alternatives

Moore, T and Stevens, G (1959) Principles of Ethics, J B Lippincott

Sampson, C (1982) The Neglected Ethic – Religious and cultural factors in the care of patients, McGraw-Hill

Thompson, I (ed) (1979) Dilemmas of Dying – A study in the ethics of terminal care, Edinburgh University Press

CHAPTER 17

THE NEEDS OF STAFF
SISTER FINBARR MALONE
and JOY ROBBINS

This chapter will consider the needs of staff, particularly nurses (both qualified and in training) when they are caring for dying patients and their families. For these purposes, nursing auxiliaries are included, since they are often involved with the care to a significant degree. Certain aspects will be intensified when such care is the nurse's exclusive function, for example in a hospice, in a continuing care unit of a hospital, or as a Macmillan nurse in the community.

However, it has already been pointed out that there are very few situations where any nurse will not sometimes be providing care during a terminal illness, however brief. It is therefore hoped that senior nurses will find the ensuing discussion helpful in considering responsibilities towards their staff, and that individual nurses will be encouraged to develop their own professional responsibility for themselves and their colleagues.

Emotional needs and support

As with many other spheres of work, terminal care carries its own type of emotional stress. The closer the relationship between nurse, patient and family, the greater is the potential strain. This should be borne in mind when allocating student nurses to care for individual patients, during one or more spans of duty. Adequate support and supervision by trained nurses should be readily available at all times, not only because the patient's condition may change quickly and unexpectedly, but to support the student emotionally.

In hospices, where it is unusual to have student nurses as part of the caring team, nursing auxiliaries often give a considerable amount of the care. They too will need careful orientation when newly appointed, continuing supervision and support from the trained nurses, and confidence that their observations and ideas are valued.

Recognizing strain

Coping with stress and anxiety is an everyday requirement for normal human growth and development (Spielberger 1979). Tolerance to stress is an individual matter; some people will exhibit strain as a response to a stressful situation very soon, whereas another person will appear not to be affected. Continuing strain is a sign that the stress being endured is excessive and can be a danger signal that actual illness will ensue.

The term 'burnout' is a recent one in this country although commonly used in the United States for a number of years. It is described as an extension of stress particularly applicable to members of the caring professions – teaching, health care, social work – when the person experiences a depletion of energy through feeling overwhelmed by other people's problems (Iveson-Iveson 1983). The person becomes increasingly fatigued, hating to go to work, and various physical symptoms may become manifest. A feeling of depression and futility is common; also headaches and sleeplessness. In desperation, even alcohol or drug dependence may start in some cases. In the place of the original high ideals and enthusiasm to serve others, a feeling of apathy and disillusion sets in, and eventually an opting-out, in a psychological if not in a physical sense, from the working group.

This tragic outcome is preventable where colleagues, and particularly those in authority, really care for each other as well as for their clients or patients. Certain personality types are more vulnerable than others, but the main factor lies in good working conditions and ready support for those helping to carry the burdens of others – often quite appalling in terms of human inadequacy and misery.

A change of job is sometimes the answer, but regrettably, talented and sensitive people are sometimes lost for ever from their chosen profession because of insufficient awareness and help from others at a crucial time.

Nursing is not exempt from this potential hazard. Those who are exclusively involved with dying and bereaved individuals should be aware of their vulnerability, and that of their colleagues; some of the ideas in this chapter may be helpful as practical measures to counterbalance the particular kind of stress involved.

Where dying people are being cared for under conditions as near as possible approaching the ideal, there is great satisfaction for the staff, compensating for the emotional stress involved. It is when there are constant anxieties and frustrations about inability to provide for a comfortable and peaceful death and continuing care for the family that the burnout syndrome is a distinct risk, especially if other factors are involved such as personal problems or a low threshold tolerance to stress.

Staff meetings

When a patient is dying, or has just died, the sharing of relevant information at a reporting session between members of the nursing staff is bound to be emotionally charged to some degree, however matter-of-factly it is conducted. This will depend on the circumstances of the patient's illness, its length, the age of the patient, and how long the individual nurses have known both patient and family. The senior nurse leading the report session should be aware that one or more nurses may be feeling particularly affected because of their closer involvement than other members of the staff.

It is important to make an opportunity for staff to talk over their own feelings, either privately with a sympathetic listener of their choice, or in a group brought together to talk over matters of mutual concern and interest outside the normal report session when time is inevitably limited because of the amount of factual information to be covered. Such a meeting can be appropriate to a general hospital ward, a hospice, a residential home for elderly people, or a home care team. It can be most valuable in bringing together members of different disciplines, each with their own expertise and problems encountered, and should promote better understanding of individual roles. Those attending should represent all those involved in caring for the dying patient, or patients, for instance all grades of nursing staff, doctors, social workers, and paramedical staff. In discussing certain matters, it will be helpful to have the psychiatrist or clinical psychologist present if such a professional worker is regularly involved.

The meeting needs an appropriate leader, who could be a member of any of the disciplines mentioned, but the atmosphere should be as relaxed as possible to encourage participation by anyone who wishes to speak. Like all meetings, if it is to be successful it should begin and end promptly at stated times and should be kept to a reasonable length. The aim of the meeting should be stated – it may be to discuss a particular patient and family because of certain problems which have arisen. Another aim might be to clarify policy on a certain issue, such as the timing of admission of a patient for terminal care. Where a patient has recently died, it may come as a relief to share feelings of doubt and anxiety as to whether the care was as adequate and well-managed as possible, and to find reassurance, or at least to admit some sense of failure and learn from it.

Good communications among staff are very important to foster appropriate attitudes. In becoming aware of the different emotional stages through which dying people and their families may pass, it becomes easier to understand that such an emotion as anger may be projected onto an individual member of staff. This may cause a natural reaction of hurt and impatient feelings in the nurse, doctor or social worker. However, in talking over the problem with others, relief is experienced that one need not feel guilty or a failure but can absorb the emotion in the team task of caring and trying to find the best way to help the patient and family. This will forestall the unfortunate sequel of the patient being avoided to some extent by some staff. Because of the variety of pressures at work, it may be difficult to hold such a meeting in a general hospital, although psychiatric hospitals will be accustomed to this means of communication. Informal exchange thus becomes very important at all levels of staff.

Working conditions

Unless the nurse is working in a hospice or other purpose-built unit, the environmental conditions may be far from ideal for the care of a dying patient. This in itself will be a strain for staff even though the patient and his family will feel more than compensated for any inconvenience of surroundings by a high quality of personal care. A major problem may be lack of a room set aside for use when privacy is essential. Doctor and ward sister frequently need to talk with close relatives, or a patient; families want to talk together and relax when spending long periods with a dying relative.

A nurse too needs some privacy during or after an emotionally traumatic time. Ingenuity can usually produce a temporary haven, and a short break away from the ward for a cup of coffee will be appreciated and enable the nurse to recover her equilibrium before resuming care of her patients.

Those nurses who are in continuous or frequent involvement with dying patients should be particularly aware of the need to balance their professional life with family, friends and recreation. Senior nurses will be mindful of the need to see that their staff have reasonable off-duty arrangements, and the occasional long break.

Professional preparation and continuing education

A nurse who chooses to work in a hospice or Macmillan service needs a thorough period of orientation and teaching in the special aspects of care. Adjustment is required from the different approach in a hospital, away from 'cure', and a trial period of employment – perhaps 3 months – is a good idea to allow for a mutual decision to be reached between the nurse and her employer that she is suited to the work. The experienced district nurse joining a Macmillan service team needs time to build up relationships with other colleagues in the community, and to learn how her special training and skills will fit into the wider team.

It may be possible for the nurse to undertake the 6-week English National Board of Nursing Studies course: 'Care of the dying patient and his family'. Otherwise, those responsible for her development in the post should see that all aspects of care are gradually learnt, building on the knowledge and experience already acquired from nursing dying patients elsewhere. Preparation of this sort is also necessary for a nurse being appointed to a unit where death frequently occurs, such as an oncological unit.

Continuing education in one's work is just as essential in terminal care as in other spheres. The responsibility for this rests with the individual nurse as well as her employers. There are regular courses and conferences arranged by hospices, by the Marie Curie Foundation, and by other bodies. The Royal College of Nursing Association of Nursing Practice has recently formed a forum – 'Symptom control and care of the dying' – open to members who are involved in such work, to provide support and educational opportunities.

There is, of course, room for multidisciplinary learning and this already takes place in many ways. A study in Scotland (Doyle 1982) into the education in terminal care received and perceived to be needed by 343 nurses reported that 87% stated a preference for multiprofessional training.

Considerable interest is shown in developing knowledge and understanding of terminal care by nurses working in areas where this is not the main feature but where the right of each individual to a peaceful and comfortable death is recognized. Study days and short conferences are always well attended, and applications to attend the longer course are numerous. This eagerness to learn how to improve patient care should result in student nurses receiving good support and teaching when they are involved in giving terminal care.

The nurse and other colleagues

In a multiprofessional setting there is always a risk that each group feels it has a monopoly of problems, so that it may not be sufficiently aware of the difficulties of other colleagues, and their needs. Some of the inadequacy of care and mismanagement of terminally ill patients – now recognized and increasingly being improved – can stem partly from lack of preparation during basic training.

Medical students can still find that low priority is given to the subject during their training. The fact that the medical student first learns the practical aspects of death in the dissecting room can lead to a defensive barrier being erected to enable the student to cope emotionally. This may affect future attitudes to dying patients. The student nurse, in contrast, is exposed at an early stage to physical and emotional contact with such patients and their families, which can help to establish more personal relationships, although of course this carries its own stress.

Other health care professional staff such as physiotherapists and occupational therapists, whose work normally has much emphasis on rehabilitation, will also need preparation for seeing the different value of their work in contributing to the comfort of the dying patient. Social workers are better equipped by their training and experience to assist patients and families emotionally, although some feel that they are not so well prepared to deal with bereaved families at home. Theological students sometimes feel that they do not have sufficient training in the practical aspects of death and bereavement for which they will later have to take responsibility – conducting funerals and facing the intense grief of relatives.

One of the nurse's functions is a co-ordinating one in the caring team. Consideration of the above factors should help in understanding and assisting colleagues who are also doing their best to help patients and their families at a critical time.

In hospices, voluntary workers give valuable help to patients and staff in a variety of ways. They too need some orientation and training in order to play their part in the service.

References

Doyle, D (1982) Nursing education in terminal care, Nursing Education Today, 2 (4), September: 4–6

Hector, W and Whitfield, S (1982) Nursing Care for the Dying Patient and the Family, William Heinemann

Iveson-Iveson, J (1983) Banishing the burnout syndrome, Nursing Mirror, May 4: 43

Popiel, E (1973) Nursing and the Process of Continuing Education, C V Mosby, St Louis

Spielberger, C (1979) Understanding Stress and Anxiety – A Life Cycle Book, Harper and Row

Thompson, I (ed) (1979) Dilemmas of Dying – A study in the ethics of terminal health care, Edinburgh University Press

Wilson-Barnet, J (1979) Stress in Hospital: Patients' psychological reactions to illness and health care, Churchill Livingstone

APPENDIX: PATIENT CARE STUDY

It seems right to finish this book with an account of a patient and her family, because many of the facets of care described in the various chapters were drawn together during the last weeks of the patient's life. The contribution has been written by a nurse who was closely involved in the caring process.

LIVING TO THE END   Sister Micheline O'Donnell

Admission and assessment

Mrs Margaret Green, a 53-year-old married lady, came to the hospice on a cold March morning from her own home, accompanied by her 23-year-old daughter, Jean. They were met at the ambulance entrance by the sister and brought to the ward. Mrs Green was to be admitted for terminal care; she had metastatic cancer of the right lung; the primary site was unknown.

Clinical picture on admission   When Mrs Green arrived at the ward she was anxious, dyspnoeic and obviously in great pain. She was made comfortable in bed and accepted a cup of tea; several of the nurses came to her bed to introduce themselves and to welcome her. Soon after this the doctor came to see Mrs Green, to take a history and to examine her with the help of a nurse. After this the doctor spent some time in just sitting with the patient and letting her talk and ask questions. She was prescribed and given an immediate dose of morphine sulphate 15 mg for relief of pain, and prochlorperazine (Stemetil) 5 mg to prevent nausea, both drugs being given orally. Mrs Green (who then asked to be called Margaret) knew her diagnosis and that she had not long to live. She said that her reason for wanting to come to the hospice was so that she could learn how to die well. She admitted that she was now feeling depressed and angry at what had happened to her. She said that at first, in the beginning of her illness, she had been told that she was imagining the pain. She had also given up a very good job. Now she just wanted 'to get it all over with'.

Family background   When the doctor was examining Margaret (as I will now call her), I sat with Jean while she had a cup of tea, and she told me about her mother and the rest of the family. Margaret's husband was aged 58 years but had to retire early because of severe rheumatoid arthritis; he walked with the aid of a stick. His wife therefore had become the family wage-earner. Their elder daughter, Pat, was 33 years old and mentally handicapped. Pat had been a source of great worry to her mother, but Jean had promised to look after her when her mother died. There was also a married son, Martin. Jean worked in a factory near home and was unmarried. The family all knew that Margaret was dying and seemed to have accepted this.

Jean also gave me the medical details which led to her mother's admission to the hospice. Margaret had been fit until 8 months previously, when she had a replacement of her left hip because of osteoarthritis. She recovered quickly from this, but on return home she developed symptoms of chest pain and dyspnoea. Unfortunately she gained the impression that the doctor thought she was imagining the pain. She then developed a pleural effusion and on X-ray metastatic lung cancer was discovered; no primary growth was found. The effusion was aspirated without relief of her symptoms. Radiotherapy was considered but not carried out, as it was thought that it would be of little or no help. Margaret was discharged home from hospital into the care of her family doctor, with the following drugs prescribed: dipipanone (Diconal) 2 tablets as required for pain; prednisolone 30 mg daily.

Nursing assessment and plan of care   The patient was in considerable pain for which a regular regimen of medication was essential. At present this could be by the oral route. Because of dyspnoea and emaciation, it would be important to try to nurse Margaret in the most comfortable position in bed or chair. Various aids to comfort should be used, also bearing in mind the risk of pressure sores occurring. Her skin was so far intact. Margaret said that her mouth was dry and that she did not feel like eating very much. These two symptoms are often related, so frequent and observant mouth care would be instituted, efforts made to stimulate her appetite, and plentiful fluids offered to her. Although there were no apparent problems at present, observation of bladder and bowel functions must be constant.

Every facility would be offered to enable the family to visit Margaret and thus help to raise her spirits. She would need to be made aware that the staff would make time to sit with her and let her talk about her feelings of anger and distress whenever she wished. It would be important to think of diversional therapy to give her satisfaction and pleasure, especially as she had always been a very active person and responsible for the welfare of her family in a very marked way.

Margaret said that she was a member of the Church of England but implied that this had been only a nominal membership for many years. However, the help of the Anglican chaplain should be offered as this is a time when people who have at least some religious beliefs may find comfort and support in renewing contact with their own faith.

Assessment of Margaret's needs would continue throughout her illness and the care being given would be regularly reviewed and changed as necessary.

It soon became evident that we must give Margaret time to come to terms with what we wished to offer her for her comfort. At first she just wanted to lie in bed with her eyes closed, remaining quite still and dreaming about dying. Jean had described her mother as stubborn and someone who usually managed to have her own way – no doubt because of the times when she had an up-hill struggle with her problems at home. We hoped to gradually help her to talk, to get the bitterness out of her system. She also needed help to live the life that was left; not just wasting the days. It was a precious time to spend with her family, whom she loved, and to do things to satisfy her active nature. The social worker called to see Margaret and to get to know her. At the moment she was not actively needed but we knew that we could call upon her at any time.

Giving care

Pain control Morphine sulphate was given 4-hourly, gradually increasing the dose until reaching 60 mg 4-hourly, which was found to control the pain completely. Prochlorperazine (Stemetil) 5 mg was given 8-hourly to prevent nausea which is often a side effect of opiate drugs. This was later changed, at Margaret's request, to metoclopramide (Maxolon) 10 mg 8-hourly. She was pleased to be able to control her drugs to a certain extent. Flurbiprofen (Froben) 100 mg twice a day was given to help the pain of bone metastases which were diagnosed soon after admission. Triazolam 0.25 mg was given at night to ensure that Margaret had a good night's sleep. Danthron (Dorbanex Forte syrup) 10 ml was given on alternate nights to counteract the constipating effect of morphine. Prednisolone 30 mg daily was given because this drug often produces an increase in appetite and a feeling of increased strength and well being. All drugs were given orally at this stage.

General hygiene and comfort Margaret liked to lie on her back all the time, so pressure area care was important. She would not lie on her side as this worsened the dyspnoea. She was supported with plenty of pillows and a sheepskin rug was placed in the bed, and later a ripple mattress. Even so, some redness appeared over the sacral area as she was very reluctant to allow her position to be changed. A daily blanket bath was given gently and without rush; any exertion increased her breathlessness. It was thought that most of the dyspnoea was caused by anxiety and so diazepam (Valium) 10 mg was prescribed and given once on several evenings. This much improved the situation together with the fact that she was free from pain.

It was while having her bath each day that Margaret talked most about her feelings. She woke up each morning disappointed that she had not died during the night. For the first few days she was still very depressed and withdrawn; when she spoke she kept her eyes closed. When her family visited her she still behaved in this way. Being the wage-earner in the family she was used to being the 'boss' – her word was law. It was difficult to persuade her to get out of bed or sit in a chair even though at this stage it would have been possible. She just wanted to lie in bed and not be disturbed. Gradually a change came in her attitude and, feeling a little better, she allowed us to take her out to the bathroom and had a bath there, which she admitted she really enjoyed. A day or two later we washed her hair, but she was always keen to go straight back to bed.

Urinary problem A week after admission to the hospice, Margaret experienced great difficulty in passing urine, her abdomen became distended, and it was eventually necessary to pass a catheter into the bladder, and commence continuous drainage. This gave her great relief until 2 days later when her urine became bloodstained and the catheter became blocked. It was removed and re-inserted. At this time the doctor wanted to give Margaret a course of antibiotics to deal with a possible urinary infection but she refused this as she thought that the treatment would prolong her life.

Mouth care   Margaret felt that her mouth was very dry and frequent glycerine of thymol mouthwashes were offered. She drank plenty of cold water which she liked, and accepted small pieces of fruit to chew.

Appetite   Margaret's appetite was poor when she first came to the hospice, but was improved to some extent by giving her small, nicely presented helpings of any food that she liked. The continuing administration of steroid drugs also helped, and gave her an improved sense of wellbeing.

Making the most of the time left

By the second week of her stay with us, Margaret began to take an interest in a number of things. She was a great music lover and started to listen to her radio again. Slowly, she began to sit out of bed for part of the day and enjoyed the nurses' coming to sit by her and talk with her. At last it seemed that she realized she was not going to die immediately and was going to live each day as it came and make the most of it. She admitted that she felt in a better frame of mind. On the first beautiful sunny day that occurred, Margaret was asked if she would like to go and see the garden. She had often told us that gardening gave her a lot of pleasure. After thinking about the suggestion for some while, Margaret got out of her dressing gown for the first time and asked for help in putting on a smart new suit that she had brought in with her. She loved the trip outside and could name every flower and shrub in the garden!

During this week the Archbishop of Canterbury had visited the hospice and had a long chat with Margaret. This had made a deep impression on her and she now attended the Anglican service in the chapel on several occasions. Margaret was now truly living to the end.

A special grief

Margaret's mother, who had been admitted to hospital about this time, was found to have cancer of the stomach and died very quickly. Margaret's son came to tell her this news. She just wanted to be on her own for a while to think about the loss of her mother. She was not well enough to attend the funeral but decided that she would spend the time in the hospice chapel instead. She was visibly upset but showed that she was also coming to terms with her own death.

Last days

From the time that she had received news of her mother's death Margaret began to deteriorate fairly rapidly. She was no longer able to get out of bed and her dyspnoea worsened again. She had become much thinner and was now only taking sips of water, but she was still able to clean her own teeth and have frequent mouthwashes. Although she was propped up in bed to help her breathlessness, she was encouraged to lie on alternate sides for short periods to prevent pressure sores forming – previous she had insisted on lying only on her back. Care of the skin continued, and attention to the urinary catheter. Her bowels did not cause much problem, and with the help of two nurses she could get out of bed to use the commode once a day. Although Margaret was now very weak, her mental outlook remained good and she knew herself that her condition was worsening.

Last 48 hours

On the 20th day of her stay in the hospice it was clear that Margaret would not live for much longer. Her husband and daughter visited her that evening and spent a long time with her. Margaret by this time was not able to talk much but knew that her family was beside her. She was no longer able to take her drugs orally so they were administered intramuscularly. She was given diamorphine 30 mg 4-hourly and metoclopramide (Maxolon) 10 mg 8-hourly, and to help her to remain tranquil chlorpromazine (Largactil) 25 mg was also prescribed 4-hourly.

Next morning Margaret's condition was worse but she was not in any distress. She knew that there was always someone near her and she occasionally mouthed a word. At mid-morning Mr Green and Jean were called to the hospice. Martin and his wife stayed at home to look after Pat. Margaret knew that they were at her bedside and seemed very peaceful and unafraid. The Anglican chaplain called and said a prayer with Margaret and the family, sitting with them for some time. He had been a regular visitor throughout her stay.

The fact that Margaret knew that they were there was a great consolation to the family. Margaret's breathing began to be noisy so hyoscine 0.4 mg was administered intramuscularly. Mr Green and Jean went for a short walk and had a cup of tea before returning to sit with Margaret again. They were offered a meal but did not feel like eating it. They were calm and accepted that Margaret would die soon. As she had been promised, Margaret was never left alone that day; a nurse would sit with her while the family had a short break. At 3 pm Margaret died very quietly and peacefully with her husband and daughter at her side. After being left together for a few minutes they were taken out to sit down and had a cup of tea with Sister and myself sitting with them. Both talked about how good a wife and mother Margaret had been, and how they would miss her. Although upset they were pleased that Margaret had died quickly in the end as she had wished. They then went home to be with Martin and his wife and Pat. After they had left, two nurses carried out Last Offices quietly and respectfully, and Margaret's body was taken to the mortuary. The family had been told that if they wished, any of them could visit the little viewing room, which is like a simple chapel, to say a last goodbye. Martin was going to see to the funeral arrangements for his father.

Evaluation
We were glad that Margaret finally reached peace and acceptance from the first feelings of anger and depression. It was felt that we had managed to control her pain and other symptoms effectively as they arose. By making the most of her last days, the family could remember her in a satisfying way, even though she had the sadness of her mother's death towards the end of her own life. The family was obviously a close one and each member would be a support to the others.

USEFUL ADDRESSES

Cruse, National Organization for the Widowed and Their Children
Cruse House
126 Sheen Road
Richmond
Surrey TW9 1UR   Tel: 01-940 4818/9047

Health Education Council
78 New Oxford Street
London WC1A 1AH   Tel: 01-637 1881

Malcolm Sargent Cancer Fund
6 Sydney Street
London SW3   Tel: 01-352 6884

Marie Curie Memorial Foundation
124 Sloane Square
London SW1X 9BP   Tel: 01-730 9157

Colostomy Welfare Group
38 Ecclestone Square
London SW1   Tel: 01-828 5175

Ileostomy Association
Amblehurst House
Chobham
Surrey   Tel: Chobham 8277

National Society for Cancer Relief
30 Dorset Square
London NW1 6QI   Tel: 01-402 8125

Society of Compassionate Friends
25 Kingsdown Parade
Bristol BS6 5UE   Tel: 0272-47316

Society for Prevention of Asbestosis & Industrial Disease
38 Drapers Road
Enfield
Middlesex   Tel: 01-366 1640

Stillbirth & Perinatal Death Association
37 Christchurch Hill
London NW3   Tel: 01-794 4601

INDEX